T0260973

TRADITIONAL CHINESE MEDICINE

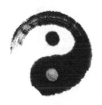

TRADITIONAL
CHINESE MEDICINE

Heritage and Adaptation

PAUL U. UNSCHULD

Translated by Bridie J. Andrews

Columbia University Press
New York

COLUMBIA
UNIVERSITY
PRESS

Columbia University Press gratefully acknowledges the generous support for this book provided by Publisher's Circle member Josephine Chiu-Duke.

Columbia University Press
Publishers Since 1893
New York   Chichester, West Sussex
cup.columbia.edu

Library of Congress Cataloging-in-Publication Data
Names: Unschuld, Paul U. (Paul Ulrich), 1943- author.
Title: Traditional Chinese medicine : heritage and adaptation / Paul U. Unschuld ; translated by Bridie J. Andrews.
Other titles: Traditionelle Chinesische Medizin. English
Description: New York : Columbia University Press, [2018] | Includes bibliographical references and index.
Identifiers: LCCN 2017021548 (print) | LCCN 2017022197 (ebook) | ISBN 9780231546263 (electronic) | ISBN 9780231175005 (cloth : alk. paper) | ISBN 9780231175012 (pbk. : alk. paper)
Subjects: | MESH: Medicine, Chinese Traditional
Classification: LCC R127.1 (ebook) | LCC R127.1 (print) | NLM WB 55.C4 | DDC 10.951—dc23
LC record available at https://lccn.loc.gov/2017021548

Cover design: Milenda Nan Ok Lee
Cover art: Chave / Jennings © Getty Images

CONTENTS

PREFACE TO THE ENGLISH EDITION

This little book was first published in German in 2013 on request by C. H. Beck. Information on Chinese medicine has been available to interested Westerners since the seventeenth century. It was only in the wake of Henry Kissinger's visit to China in 1971 that the modernized version of historical Chinese medicine, so-called Traditional Chinese Medicine (TCM), gained worldwide attention. Since then, there is hardly a small town, not to speak of major cities, in Europe or the United States where no TCM is offered. Clinics have been opened by a most heterogeneous group of practitioners. These may be Chinese citizens with or without prior health care experience in their own country; Korean, Vietnamese, and Japanese migrants; Europeans; or U.S. citizens. They all claim to practice TCM, and yet their educational backgrounds and their competence in acupuncture and Chinese pharmaceutics, massage, dietetics, and other therapeutic approaches differ considerably. Germany, for example, has had a rather multicultural therapy system for centuries. Modern biomedicine may dominate, but Germany's own historical therapeutic heritage has remained lively and sought after by many. Hence it is not a clear-cut antagonism between Western and Chinese medicine that has emerged since the opening of China.

Rather, Chinese medicine has joined an already colorful health care scenario. The problem is, hardly anybody in health politics circles knew how to deal with this new arrival. So many questions emerged. How should a practitioner's competence be assessed? What is the role of historical Chinese theoretical foundations, such as the yin-yang and Five Phases theories? How much of these foundations are required to practice acupuncture and Chinese pharmaceutical therapy? Why was Chinese medicine defamed by virtually all reformers in the first half of the twentieth century? Has Chinese medicine been a stable system of theory and practice since ancient times, as some claim, or has it been subject to constant modification and renewal based on new insights of practitioners and natural scientists? And, quite significantly, will TCM and Western medicine be contradictory approaches to maintaining health and curing disease forever, or will the two eventually merge into one type of medicine that is superior to its two parents?

These are some of the many questions raised over the past three to four decades. The arrival of TCM in other countries of the Western world poses a public health problem. To solve it, decision makers and the general public need solid information. To take a close look at the history of Chinese medicine and to make available reliable data on its many facets is a challenge I have aimed at responding to ever since the beginnings of my academic career in the Departments of Behavioral Sciences and International Health at the Johns Hopkins School of Hygiene and Public Health in Baltimore in 1980. There I taught courses on "Problems associated with the introduction of Western medicine into societies with traditional medical systems of their own." Now the situation has reversed: a foreign traditional medical system is being introduced into virtually all Western health care delivery systems. With this background I began, decades ago, to translate ancient Chinese medical core texts into English in order to offer insights into the beginnings of Chinese medicine. Too little was known in the 1970s and subsequent years on the history of Chinese pharmaceutical lore, Chinese medical ethics, etc. It is very comforting to see how research and publications on these and other issues have expanded in recent years.

The present book offers a concise summary of the history of medicine in China, its close connection with Chinese culture in general and with Chinese politics in particular. It compares basic features of historical Chinese medicine with historical European/Western medicine and shows the departure of TCM from its historical origins. The fall of the Chinese Empire in 1911 and China's subsequent quest to regain its former strength by learning from the West and then linking that knowledge with its own cultural assets has deeply influenced the nature of Chinese medicine, resulting in TCM. Recently, a Nobel Prize in Physiology or Medicine has been awarded to a Chinese researcher, the pharmacologist Tu Youyou. This extraordinary valuation has given new impetus to a debate that never really ended in modern China, about the place of tradition in a society that aims to be the most creative industrial nation worldwide by 2049, one hundred years after the founding of the People's Republic of China. In December 2016, China's top legislature, the National People's Congress Standing Committee, passed a law on Traditional Chinese Medicine, giving TCM a bigger role in the medical system The law went into effect on July 1, 2017. In 1915, Japan attempted to impose on China twenty-one conditions of military, economic, and political dependence. One century after this most painful humiliation, marking the apex of intrusions by foreign powers into Chinese territory and sovereignty, China feels strong enough again to reconsider its own cultural, scientific, technological, and medical heritage. I wrote this book to help readers in the United States and beyond to understand the changing Chinese attitudes toward Chinese medicine and develop a suitable reaction to the opening of this health care tradition to the entire world.

Paul U. Unschuld
Berlin, January 2017

TRADITIONAL CHINESE MEDICINE

INTRODUCTION

Information about a specifically Chinese art of healing first arrived in Europe from East Asia in the late sixteenth century. Portuguese Jesuit priests working in Japan were the first to report to their superiors about a remarkable new method, unknown in their native land, of introducing thin needles through the skin into the body tissues of sick patients in order to achieve therapeutic effects. In the following centuries, doctors were able to travel first to Southeast Asia and then to China proper, initially with the Dutch East India Company, then with the British, and lastly in the service of various American missionary societies. There they witnessed Chinese needle therapy firsthand, and they named it with the Latin term *acupunctura*, or "puncturing with sharp objects." The English word "acupuncture" is derived from this. They also reported on other healing methods, particularly Chinese herbal medicine and the burning of small quantities of dried herbs on particular skin locations to influence the condition of the human organism. The Japanese word for burning, *mokusa*, and its Latin equivalent were combined in the creation of the new English term "moxibustion."

Nowadays, what is called Traditional Chinese Medicine, or TCM for short, is well known throughout the Western world as a contribution from Chinese cultural history to the modern healing landscape. There is no other field in which modern China could have attracted so much appreciative attention for its historical cultural creativity. No other aspect of the two-and-a-half-thousand-year prehistory of modern China has left such a simultaneously deep and positive impression on the scientifically and technologically sophisticated populations of industrial nations as has TCM. This is an astonishing phenomenon when considered in the context of the enormous recent diagnostic and therapeutic achievements of Western medicine, which were scarcely imaginable only a few decades ago. How has such an unproven and scientifically unverifiable set of ancient and foreign healing methods been able to arouse such great interest among Western industrial nations, to the point where it must be considered a serious component of their health care systems?

Not only laypeople and fringe healers are motivated to study and use acupuncture and traditional Chinese pharmaceuticals. Many physicians, after successfully completing their lengthy courses of study at the medical schools of European and North American universities, all devoted exclusively to Western science and the diagnostic and therapeutic principles derived from it, have turned to non-European healing traditions to look for effective treatment methods. And many have had their expectations confirmed. Among such foreign healing traditions, Traditional Chinese Medicine occupies one of the most prominent positions, alongside Ayurveda from India.

The purpose of this book is to explore the historical origins of this phenomenon and to describe and interpret its contemporary significance.

The first section is devoted to the emergence of a recognizably Chinese medicine more than two thousand years ago, beginning in the second century before the Common Era. It indicates how the radical political changes occurring toward the end of the Zhou era (1046–256 B.C.E.) and during the Qin dynasty (221–206 B.C.E.), and culminating in the Han dynasties (lasting from 206 B.C.E. to 8 C.E. and from 23 to 219 C.E.), stimulated new ways of thinking. These not only brought forth a new vision of society but also stimulated the development of a new worldview that included a completely novel understanding of the human organism in health and disease. The methods of prevention and cure that were derived from this new understanding are what we refer to today as historical Chinese medicine. The ancient texts that document this medicine are still available, even though they are preserved in editions dating from later centuries. They are still consulted by advocates for the clinical relevance of Traditional Chinese Medicine and are considered part of the foundation of their practice.

The second part considers the development of Chinese medicine and its global distribution in the form of Traditional Chinese Medicine from about the beginning of the nineteenth century, paying particular attention to recent events in China and Europe. Up until the nineteenth century, European physicians were generally very open to new ideas from foreign cultures. Reports from China describing comparatively very different ways of dealing with disease were enthusiastically received at a time when European doctors were deeply insecure about their own medical knowledge. European medicine was still searching for a paradigm that would eventually assimilate the many new discoveries about human morphology and physiology and then, in short order, combine them with the recently published advances in chemistry, physics, and their associated technologies into a convincing theoretical superstructure. Such a comprehensive synthesis was achieved for the first time in the middle of the nineteenth century with the theories of cellular physiology and pathology of Rudolph Virchow (1821–1902).

In the eighteenth century, reports of Chinese needle therapies were combined with the new understanding of electricity, and needles were interpreted as potential stimulators of the body's own electrical power. The result was described by one early nineteenth-century doctor as a widespread "acupuncture mania" in Europe— at the same time as acupuncture was being removed from the curriculum of the Chinese Imperial Medical Academy, banned as a practice within the Forbidden City, and coming under increasing criticism in China, its place of origin.

The rise of modern Western medicine from about 1835 and the concomitant awakening of a new self-confidence on the part of its physicians and scientists led to a rapid decline of interest in Chinese medicine. After 1850, acupuncture and other Chinese healing methods were known to only a few; they played no further detectable role in public discourse or in clinical practice. How it came to be that TCM is again a generally recognized term, with tens of thousands of doctors and healers in Western industrialized nations claiming to have successfully treated many satisfied patients, is a development that still requires explanation and investigation.

In the opposite direction, European-American medicine, which became known simply as "Western medicine," found ready acceptance and was quickly disseminated in China after the middle of the nineteenth century. At that time, the European powers, followed by the United States and then finally China's neighbor Japan, imposed a series of humiliating military defeats on China, which had long considered itself the "Middle Kingdom." This caused Chinese reformers and revolutionaries to doubt the validity of both their own sciences and their medical tradition. They decided that only the wholesale adoption of Western medicine could guarantee an effective health care system appropriate for the construction of a "new China." It would be decades after the founding of the People's Republic of China in 1949, after its opening to the West in the

1970s, before the Chinese side would recognize the global economic potential of marketing their newly modernized "traditional" medicine.

A contradiction has developed between the widespread desire in Western industrialized nations to use "Traditional Chinese Medicine" as an example of a physical and spiritual alternative to "Western medicine" and the official Chinese policy of integrating this same TCM into the biomedical explanatory framework of Western medicine, particularly the desire to market Chinese-style pharmaceuticals worldwide after they are legitimated according to the most up-to-date biological criteria. This contradiction extends its influence beyond the present, and will continue to influence the future dynamics of TCM.

I

THE HISTORICAL FOUNDATIONS

1

ORIGINS AND CHARACTERISTICS
OF CHINESE MEDICINE

In 221 B.C.E., Ying Zheng, the king of Qin, brought a centuries-long period of warfare among multiple smaller states (an era known to history as the Warring States period) to an end. After long years of successful military campaigns, he was able to consolidate power and declare himself "First Emperor of Qin."[1] Qin Shi Huang Di, as he is known in Chinese, became in that moment the architect of the political structure of imperial China, a structure that has lasted longer than any other in world history. Not until 2,133 years later did a Manchu ruler by the name of Aisin-Gioro Pu Yi became the last of Qin Shi Huang Di's successors by abdicating in January 1912. A few weeks earlier, in October 1911, the new Republic of China had been declared.

The success of the First Emperor in eliminating, with great ruthlessness, the last six states that were competing with Qin for supremacy earned Qin Shi Huang Di an outstanding position in Chinese historiography. His tomb, where he had himself buried along with thousands of individually fashioned, life-size terracotta warriors, has made him famous throughout the modern world since its discovery and opening to tourism in the 1970s.

Qin Shi Huang Di is unlikely to have wasted much thought on the development of Chinese medicine. However, the new political structures that he created and left behind (after less than two decades at the helm of the newly united Chinese state) became so deeply imprinted in the consciousness of many of the intellectual elites of the time that they even influenced their interpretation of the structures of the human body—the body was modeled on the state. Efforts to keep the body healthy and to combat disease were expected to follow the same principles as the pacification of society. Observers of the state and of the human body at this time saw no difference in approach to these two realms: indeed, the same word, *zhi* 治, which has a general meaning of "to put in order," was used to indicate both ruling (the state) and treating (a person).

By the third century B.C.E., China had already achieved a high degree of cultural civilization. The writing system had been perfected and was designed to express highly sophisticated political, philosophical, and military concepts and ideas. The thousands of characters gave educated authors the ability to fully express themselves in writing. A network of educated readers, dispersed over great geographical distances, created a need for these manuscripts, which were repeatedly copied as they made their way to their recipients. The First Emperor retained the most talented advisors to help create, in short order, an integrated economic and cultural organism out of the final seven territories. As a result of his standardization of weights, measures, written characters, and road and axle widths, along with other initiatives, it became possible to establish large cities, which had in turn to be supplied from distant hinterlands. The unimpeded circulation of people and goods was the precondition for the maintenance of the new political order.

At that time, people were still living under the trauma of the previous centuries. Contemporary observers complained that all moral sensibility had been lost in the years of indiscriminate conflict. The unification of the country had been achieved by using weapons to end the wars between individual states, but the trauma of internecine conflict remained; it can still be found today in the Chinese collective mentality. The lesson of the preceding centuries was that it is not the good but the cunning who survive. This encouragement to deploy whatever crafty strategies might give an advantage in the ongoing struggle for survival can still be found in the cultural heritage of modern China.[2]

2

THE LACK OF
EXISTENTIAL AUTONOMY

In those days, survival was clearly not only a matter of avoiding the human enemies who came to take one's land, property, and more. A person's life was also threatened by invisible forces that, like human enemies, were lurking everywhere and had to be warded off. The conclusion for people of the time—and for the majority of the Chinese people until very recent times—was that it was almost impossible to be in control of your own life. The length and quality of one's earthly existence depended on forces over which humans had only uncertain influence. Whether and when you might become ill or even die of illness was out of your own hands. The forces that controlled such matters could, at best, be beseeched or placated with offerings.

In this period, when the king of Qin was declaring himself the divinely appointed First Emperor of China, people who wondered about the causes of ill health and early death knew who exercised power over this earthly life. They had identified various forces to which they could ascribe the sufferings that haunted them. Ancestors had particular significance in the causation of disease. As early as about 1000 B.C.E., ox scapulae and tortoise plastrons (the underparts of tortoise shells) were used as divination devices by the living to ask the dead about the cause of the wrath of an ancestor and hence the illness of a descendant, and whether an offering, in the form of a sacrifice, would appease it.

Concepts of the relationship between the living and the dead became increasingly sophisticated. The idea that ancestors would punish their living descendants for their sins evolved in the course of the centuries into the idea that living descendants would have to bear the punishments for the past sins of their ancestors as well as for their own transgressions. Certainly by the time of the Han dynasty, and possibly as early as the Shang, it was agreed there were nine generations of ancestors still active in the afterlife. They were held to account for all the offenses they had committed while alive, and every indictment in the underworld led to an illness among their living descendants.

From this perspective, the efforts of the living to protect their own health became insignificant. People lived with the feeling of complete inability to influence the conditions of their existence. On the many bronze vessels found buried in Shang-dynasty tombs, we often find inscriptions that effusively praise the individuals they accompanied into the afterlife. It is possible that these glorifications were intended as testimony to be placed before the judge of the underworld, to be weighed against the crimes of the deceased, not least out of the self-interest of the survivors, who would otherwise bear the brunt of any punishment.

The ancestors were not the only spirits who could make things difficult for the living. Beginning in the Warring States period, the ancestors had competition in the form of demons. Demons were not identified by their family connections to the living, but rather, having died an unnatural or violent death, bore a grudge against all of humanity. They expressed this resentment by causing all kinds of malicious damage. The only thing the people of the Warring States knew to use against such spirits was violence, of the form they had learned to use against their human enemies. Resistance could be initiated through an alliance with a powerful deity, such as the sun, the moon, or the stars, or through the invocation of particularly powerful spirits who were known to specialize in devouring lower-ranked demonic beings.

The creativity the early Chinese brought to devising words, gestures, objects, and substances to reflect the increasing diversity of concepts, such as how evil spirits caused harm and how most effectively to protect oneself from them, has continued largely unabated into the present. These ideas are clearly further evidence of their underlying sense of existential uncertainty: the knowledge that the quality and length of human life largely depended on forces that the living could only imperfectly resist, and then only with great effort.

"Heaven," regarded as an abstract being, was also considered responsible for human fate. Long before the title *di* 帝, divine ruler, was secularized and applied to a human, the label "Heaven" referred to a deity who was conceptually far less anthropomorphic than anything in the Judeo-Christian West. That is why we find in the Confucian *Analects* the saying "Life and death are governed by fate, wealth and honor are determined by Heaven."[1] Humans had no influence over Heaven, so the existential uncertainty not only applied to the influence of ancestors, ghosts, and demons but also extended to such abstract forces.

The many initiatives that people in ancient times took to protect their lives by appeasing the ancestors, demons, and Heaven seemed to be effective often enough to consolidate belief in these forms of existence. The *Book of Songs* 詩經, a text most probably compiled in the late Zhou dynasty, records many instances of using specific modes of communication with the spirit world to good effect. Ultimately, ghosts were still (faded) persons, even if some of them were particularly malevolent:

Their spirits happily enjoy the offerings of food and drink, and in return, will cause you to live long.[2]

When the forms and rituals are according to rule, and smiles and speaking are appropriate, the spirits come and reciprocate with great blessings. Ten thousand years are the reward.[3]

Even today, when unprovable kinds of faith healing seem to yield the desired results, many people evaluate them with the sentence "Whatever works is right." The exact same logic has been at work across the entire period from more than two thousand years ago until today: those who were able to demonstrate success with their incantations and exorcisms felt vindicated by the results. Their demonstrations of success provided justification not only for their methods but also, above all, for the theories that undergirded them. The belief system of antiquity was coherent but not comforting, because the forces that negatively influenced human life were arbitrary and unpredictable. This arbitrariness, referred to in modern theological circles as "God's inscrutability," was already described in the *Book of Songs*. We see it in the still powerful lament of a desperate man who had tried all possible means to procure relief: "The drought is endless, the shimmering heat is agonizing. I have offered up pure sacrifices without ceasing. . . . There is no spirit I have not honored."[4] No reaction occurred, and nobody was able to explain why.

3

THE LONGING FOR
EXISTENTIAL AUTONOMY

It is necessary to retain an acute awareness of this basic sense that life was dependent on scarcely controllable forces to truly appreciate how disorienting was the revolution in thinking expressed in the new and completely oppositional worldview that accompanied the unification of the state. We find the rationale for the change expressed only much later by various authors, such as Ge Hong, ca. 280–340 C.E., and Tao Hongjing, 456–536 C.E., who declared: "My fate lies in my own hands, not in Heaven!" (*Wo ming zi wo bu zai tian* 我命在我不在天). With this, they were uttering the same longing for existential autonomy that had already been expressed several centuries earlier in a much more formal sense in the new medicine, as they were well aware.

As always, when a fundamental theoretical innovation is introduced into the history of medicine, we must ask when considering its origins, why did it occur in this way, and why at that particular time? So we will first consider the characteristics of the new medicine.

Underlying the new perspective on the human organism in conditions of health and sickness was a concerted effort to reject the superior power of the spirits, including Heaven. One could have simply negated them: they don't exist! But that would have been a mistake. Our own recent history shows that when one wants to erase a concept from people's consciousness, one should not avoid the word that expresses the concept. On the contrary, one should retain the word and redefine it with completely new and opposing content. This was the case with the early Marxists, who had no use for the word "freedom" in its conventional sense, so they redefined it—"freedom is the recognition of necessity"— thereby turning it into its opposite. Necessity was to be determined by the Communist Party.[1]

A similar procedure occurred when the small band of philosophers known as the Yin-Yang School sought to free themselves from the power of the spirits. They retained the word for spirits or deities, *shen* 神, and redefined it in two different ways. First, the spirits were newly identified, no longer as invisible beings in the human environment but rather as the concrete substances, blood and *qi*, that were necessary for human life: "Blood and *qi* are the spirits within humans. One must nourish them carefully!"[2] The literal translation of the character *qi* is "steam rising from rice." The original meaning included both the breath and the gases that escape as a result of digestion, as well as the supposed currents of vapors that, like the blood, flowed throughout the organism and whose obstruction, counterflow, or excessive discharge could lead to disease. In the following centuries, the word *qi* was invested with various new meanings, so that it is not possible to translate it one-to-one with any single appropriate word in a European language.

A second reinterpretation of the spirits was to prove substantially more effective. From now on, the spirits would no longer have power over humans. On the contrary: humans had power over the spirits. The new medicine provided an explanation for this: within the human organism, attached to one or more organs, is a spirit. The Chinese character for such organs is *zang* 藏, which means long-term depot, or in this context, long-term storage organs. In other words, long-term depots are where important goods are protected for extended periods. There is another category of organ in the body, the *fu* 府 or short-term repositories. There are no spirits trapped in these organs. They take in goods one day and release them again the next day, if not before. The spirits are retained securely within the body as long as the long-term storage organs have sufficient reserves of *qi*. Each organ has a natural endowment of healthy *qi*, but if this is carelessly overspent, it may become insufficient to retain the organ spirit. In that case, the spirit frees itself, with all kinds of negative consequences for the human host.

It is therefore within each person's power to control these spirits within the body or to let them escape. Control operates through the emotions. An undisciplined approach to one's own emotions will quickly use up the resources of whichever long-term storage organs are responsible for maintaining those emotions. Thus emotions are the only internal causes of the exhaustion of the body's organic resources, the displacement of the internal spirits, and the vulnerability that allows external pathogens to implant themselves in the body, resulting in all kinds of diseases. When some East Asians today give the impression of being better able to quell their emotions than many Europeans, it is due to the enduring effects of this ancient Chinese theory about the intimate causes of disease. For two thousand years, until the encounter with European medicine, this theory determined the culture of at least the educated elites.

This theory of the localization of spirits in the organs is not just important for understanding ancient Chinese medicine and the alternating power relationships between humans and spirits: it also highlights the traumatic effects of the previous hundreds of years of conflict. The resources of the long-term storage organs may be "replete" (*shi* 實) or "depleted" (*xu* 虛). But "replete" does not refer to a healthy, normal state, which was described differently. An emptiness or "depletion" occurs when the resources are used up. A long-term storage organ is then no longer able to perform its various functions. So, for example, a healthy gleam in the eyes depends on there being sufficient resources in the liver. A lack of these resources also indicates a much more serious danger, as suggested by the memory of the Warring States period. The depletion of a long-term depot in the human body is analogous to a breach in the walls of a city or a weakening of the defenses of the state. It allows neighbors or foreign states who learn of it to take immediate advantage, invading and lodging in places where they don't belong. This is what is meant by "full" or "replete."

The world is organized according to two categories: the proper, orthodox, or correct, *zheng* 正 on the one hand, and the evil, improper, heterodox, or aberrant *xie* 邪 on the other. There is no middle ground. Wind, cold, dampness, and other natural conditions are basically normal. Without moisture, the fields would not yield their harvests, and without the wind, the damp earth would never dry out. But if wind or dampness takes advantage of the depletion of an organ to invade the human body and cause all kinds of pathological processes, then the formerly "correct" state of these natural phenomena has become "evil," and it is necessary to root them out. The new medicine promised to show people how to behave so that they would be able to maintain their health and also to correct any incipient depletion or repletion. This corresponds to the two kinds of behavior in society: the correct or upright and the evil, incorrect, or aberrant. Good and evil are not absolute categories that can be ascribed to things or people. Rather, whoever keeps their place and does their duty is "upright." Whoever leaves their ascribed role or position and trespasses where they do not belong, in doing so becomes "evil." The presence of this "evil" in the body is disease.

4

QUOTATIONS FROM THE
MEDICAL CLASSICS

Let us consider some quotations from the oldest known medical text, the "Plain Questions" edition of the *Yellow Emperor's Inner Classic* (*Huang Di nei jing su wen*). They illustrate both the new understanding of health and disease and how to protect the body as the first priority and treat it when protection fails, all in the idiom of the ancient authors. The *Huang Di nei jing su wen* was compiled in the first or second century C.E. by unknown editors from a variety of texts and text fragments from equally anonymous authors who wrote from the second century B.C.E. on. Most of the texts were constructed by the compilers as a dialogue between the Yellow Emperor and Qi Bo, an interlocutor whose name is not found in any previous literature.

According to this structure, Huang Di, the Yellow Emperor, is the questioner, the one who seeks knowledge. Qi Bo is the educator, the learned one. At times the dialogue descends into crude rebukes by the teacher of the questioner's ignorance. Who can have come up with this idea of allowing such a nobody to behave so disrespectfully toward the mythic Yellow Emperor, one of the most revered founding heroes of Chinese culture?

It may be that the name Qi Bo is a faint echo of the name Hippo[crates], whose reputation as the founder of ancient Greek medicine had quite possibly already spread far beyond the borders of the eastern Mediterranean and the ancient Middle East. Conceivably his fame had reached as far as East Asia and inspired the compilers of the *Huang Di nei jing su wen* to adopt this remarkable form of dialogue. It is also noticeable that the editors, while reorganizing the many original texts, often inserted key sayings at the beginning or end of each chapter, whose validity extended further than the merely medical. This is where the relationship between specific healing concepts and the higher-level sociopolitical realm is spelled out explicitly. "Evil accumulates where there is lack of *qi*"[1] is a clear indication of the duty everyone has to conserve their own natural endowment of *qi*. "When essence and spirit are conserved within, where can disease arise from?"[2]

The concept of an "essence" in the body was an attempt to create terminological distance from the close relationship of the word "spirit" (*shen* 神) with the earlier concepts of ancestors and demons, and to postulate a material substrate, an "essence" (*jing* 精), as the basis of bodily vitality. "Essence" and "spirit" are often linked in a compound word, or are used singly and interchangeably. The phrase "essence and spirit" could also be expressed as "essence-spirit." The author of this quotation was in any case certain that essence and spirit, or essence-spirit, were under the control of every individual person. One's behavior determined whether the spirit was able to extract itself from control. And the correct way to behave is clearly and repeatedly explained in the *Huang Di nei jing su wen*: "Obedience leads to alignment. Without [obedience], there will be counteralignment. Where there is counteralignment, changes are generated, and changes lead to disease."[3]

The question remains, to what requirements, standards, or even laws does this demand for obedience refer? The new medical reasoning leaves no room for misunderstanding here, either. Heaven is now merely the "great emptiness" that covers the earth. Humans stand on the earth and under heaven, which is no longer considered capable of exerting a numinous power over human fate. Instead, heaven and earth are no more and no less than the natural sources of *qi* that nature makes available to all humans. Birth, maturation, and death are determined no longer by the unfathomable whims of Heaven as abstract supernatural being, but rather by the course of nature, which is expressed most visibly in the progression of the seasons: "[Protected by the] canopy of heaven and supported by the earth, the myriad beings come into existence. Nothing is nobler than humanity. Humans receive life from the *qi* of heaven and earth, and mature according to the law of the four seasons."[4]

The first thing to notice here is the preeminent position ascribed to humanity. Mankind is denoted as the noblest of beings—so how can it also be the plaything of various numinous powers? The central point in this quote is clearly the word "law," *fa* 法. This word was multivalent in ancient Chinese, and had the additional meanings of criminal law; model, pattern, or standard; and method. There were no previous classical texts that would support an interpretation of *fa* as "natural law," however. That was new. Nature was now seen as following the Way, *dao* 道, with a regularity that made it a model for humanity. If humans conformed to these secular regularities, or laws, all would go well for them: "If the Way is carefully observed in accordance with the law, . . . the Mandate of Heaven will last long."[5]

It was not Heaven that gave or took the Mandate that determined the life or death of humans. They could decide for themselves how long and how well to live. As stated in the slogan recorded by both Ge Hong (ca. 280–ca. 340 C.E.) and Tao Hongjing (456–536), "My fate lies in my own hands, not in Heaven!", for a group of Chinese observers of nature, the power of supernatural forces had long been broken. Ge Hong's alchemical efforts to find an elixir of eternal life arose out of this consciousness of human agency. The editors of one passage in the *Huang Di nei jing su wen* were so eager to promote their belief as an all-encompassing law that they repeatedly inserted the formula "The same law above and below" in a staccato fashion and without regard to its relationship with the rest of the text.[6]

The dread and terror of arbitrary punishments by ancestors or spirits was replaced in this new mindset with punishments that were inflicted automatically—and that was the difference—whenever the laws of nature were violated. "Minor [transgressions] are met by slight revenge. Severe [transgressions] are met by severe revenge. That is the regularity of *qi*."[7]

Qi, we should note, was something entirely material, unrelated to ancestors or demons.

5

THE BANALITY OF VIOLENCE

The assertion that there was an invisible law behind the patterns and regularities observable in nature provided a foundation for the development of an entirely secular science, just as had been the case only a few centuries earlier in the eastern Mediterranean. In ancient Greece the questions of analysis concentrated on the basic structures of objects and of life, but in China, despite similar initial investigations into these basic structures, the investigative project went down a different path. The relational cosmology that had been developed to only a limited extent in Europe and then overlooked in favor of analytical science took precedence in China and, in the theories of yin-yang and the Five Phases of all natural beings, remained constitutive of Chinese culture for more than two thousand years.

Relational cosmology proceeds from the assumption that all phenomena, tangible or intangible, may be organized according to a limited number of categories. In yin-yang theory, there may be two, four, six, or twelve such categories; in Five Phases theory, there are five. Phenomena grouped into any one category are similar in nature. In their relationships to phenomena of other categories, they behave according to the regular patterns of relationships between the various groups of two, four, six, twelve, or five, respectively. Understanding the commonalities of phenomena in a particular category and the relationships between the categories allowed a person to understand the processes of creation, growth, maturation, and dying, and to orient his or her life accordingly.

These theories illuminate once again the traumatic effects of the Warring States period. Both the yin-yang theory and the Five Phases theory reflect a worldview in which violence—destruction, domination, retaliation, and revenge—was the norm. This basic understanding of the warlike past was corroborated in nature. Every day, the darkness obliterated the light. Yet no sooner had the darkness achieved dominance than the light began its retaliation and destroyed it again. The progression of the seasons, the rise and fall of dynasties—wherever one looked, violence was the natural order of things. By formulating their observations of nature in terms of the theories of yin-yang and the Five Phases, intellectuals were recognizing the normality of persistent violence: "When the *qi* dominate each other, then there is harmony. If there is no mutual domination, then there is disease."[1] These theories provided the knowledge needed to survive in this environment: "Understanding the cycle of conquering and retaliation is the model for all of humanity. It demonstrates the Way of Heaven."[2]

The downside of this new view of human life, the price of this existential autonomy, was great. Suffering humanity now had no one to blame but itself for its troubles. The same ice-cold indifference of the Legalist and Confucian social theories, and later also of Buddhism after its adoption from India, all insisting on the importance of individual responsibility, was characteristic of ancient Chinese medicine. The rules of survival and the guidelines that one had to follow were known to all. Whoever adapted to them survived, while those who disobeyed suffered the consequences. So it is not surprising that the body itself was interpreted according to this new way of thinking and constituted as a governable organism; after all, the preservation of the body is medicine's primary duty.

6

THE MAWANGDUI TEXTS

Since the 1970s, many new archaeological discoveries have transformed our understanding of the origins and early history of Chinese medicine. The so-called Mawangdui manuscripts, from an excavated tomb near Changsha, the capital of Hunan province, and dated near the beginning of the second century B.C.E., were the first evidence of the state of Chinese healing arts before the creation of the new medicine that relied only on the secular laws of nature. Similar texts from around 200 B.C.E. were discovered in other gravesites far from Mawangdui. All of them offer insight into the theoretical and practical healing methods of the literate elites of that time. Noticeably, they contain no mention of the theories of yin-yang and Five Phases found in the new medicine of only a century later. Yin and yang were merely used as markers for pairs of opposites. There is also no mention of acupuncture in these texts.

Spirits were blamed as the perpetrators of diseases; injuries came from animals or as the result of accidents. From this theoretical standpoint it was necessary to exorcise the disease-causing demons with spoken spells, specific gestures, and the administration of medications. The texts also contain illustrations of gymnastic breathing exercises. Sexual practices for the maintenance of health are described alongside the criteria for differentiating curable patients from the incurable. As was the case everywhere in the ancient world, it was not advisable for a doctor to tend to the latter. Any doctor who tended to a patient whose disease proved fatal was considered incompetent and was likely to suffer social and legal sanctions. This led to a great deal of attention being paid to prognostication, the ability to predict the future development of a disease.

When we compare the healing arts of the Mawangdui texts with the medicine developed only slightly later, there are several significant differences. First is the absence of any description of the natural laws humans must adhere to if they wish to remain healthy. Second is the spectacular nature of the medications. There are more than two hundred recipes describing a similar number of natural substances for pharmaceutical use in the treatment of various internal and external diseases. These substances were prepared into raw drug form using pharmaceutical technologies that were clearly very elaborate, then further processed into different forms for administration, such as pills or decoction, depending on their intended therapeutic purpose. This rich pharmaceutics appears to the modern observer as already in a highly developed state; there are no known sources describing how it might have developed gradually over time.

On the other hand, the texts' descriptions of the structure of the human body and its manifestations of disease are important in elucidating how the documented views of Chinese medical authors changed in the short span of a century between the Mawangdui texts and the medicine of the Han dynasty. The earlier medical observers imagined a total of eleven single, unconnected conduits containing *qi*, i.e., vapors, and blood that could be stirred by stimulation into movement. These movements could be detected with the fingers at various points on the body—thus describing the beginnings of pulse diagnosis, which was to become such an important element of diagnostics later in Chinese medicine. Each conduit had a beginning and an end, and they extended through the limbs, the torso, and the head. The movements of their contents could lead to various kinds of discomfort along the paths of the conduits. Additionally, the Mawangdui texts described three internal organs, without mention of any relationship to the eleven individual conduits.

7

ANATOMY, PHYSIOLOGY, AND PATHOLOGY IN THE NEW MEDICINE

The creators of the new medicine certainly knew what the insides of a human, or at least an animal, body looked like when examined by someone without medical knowledge. They, however, were able to see more than any untrained observer. In the human body, they discerned a reflection of the society in which they lived. The individual organs were organized into an administrative hierarchy. They were referred to by the same bureaucratic titles as their counterparts in the state administration. From ruler down to the administrators responsible for transportation, food storage, and even censorship, each found its equivalent in the human body. Various models of this emerged at around the same time, but all conveyed the same message: the human body has the same basic structure as the unified empire. Five formerly unconnected "administrative centers," the lungs, heart, spleen, liver, and kidneys, were now conceived as linked together into an integrated whole through a complex system of transportation routes. This new view described the governors who ruled over each of these "administrative centers" and also the subordinates who were subject to their rule: the blood was ruled by the heart and resided in the "palace" of the small intestine; the bones and sinews were ruled by the kidneys and resided in the bladder "palace," and so on. One can still detect in the ancient formulations of the authors of this system their conviction that each of the "administrative centers" would take advantage of a weakness in its neighbors to immediately mount an invasion. The terminology reflected this translation of hundreds of years of experience into the physiological processes of the human organism.

Because every one of the authors who contributed to this new concept of the human body was convinced of the validity of yin-yang theory, they naturally saw yin-yang duality in the inner and outer aspects of the body. The twofold division of organs into five long-term and six short-term storage organs (*wu zang* 五藏 and *liu fu* 六府) represents only one of the consequent pairings. The human organism, like the state, possessed defense forces. Yin-yang theory brought the certainty that there must be both yin and yang defenses. The first of these, corresponding to yin, were stationary; the new observers chose to represent them with the term *ying* 營, stationary garrison, military camp. The second, corresponding to yang, were mobile. They were represented in the new medical terminology by the term *wei* 衛, or mobile sentries, guardians. Shortly thereafter, these observers recognized that the back of the body, its yang surface, and the breast and belly area of the body, its yin surface, each exhibited a straight, unbranched conduit that led from the top of the body to the bottom. Accordingly, they designated the yang conduit as the controller vessel (*ren mai* 任脈), named after the mobile officials who traveled from place to place to exert their controlling function. The yin conduit on the belly side was the supervisor vessel (*du mai* 督脈), named after the stationary officials who sat in their offices to exercise their supervisory functions.

The insides of the body were filled with "warp threads," *jing* 經. They constituted a circulatory system, one each on the left, or yang, and right, or yin, side of the body. The "warp threads" were thought of not as actual threads, but rather channels through which blood and *qi* flowed. These channels were considered as important for the human organism as warp threads are for a textile—hence the metaphor. If a warp thread ruptures, then the textile falls apart. The conduits in the body had the same functions as the network of transportation routes in the newly unified empire. They connected the formerly isolated administrative centers. Their contents flowed sometimes in one direction, sometimes in the other. The medical experts detected currents that flowed in different directions within the same conduit, just as occurred on the busy roads. On different stretches of the conduit, the proportions of blood and *qi* might vary considerably, presenting the possibility of congestion and as a result, pain.

Traffic in the body's internal conduits was also affected by atmospheric conditions. Different rules applied in summer than in winter. The daytime currents were different from the flows at night. It was therefore necessary to take these traffic variations into account in order to maintain well-being in spite of the changing physiological and pathological conditions of the body that accompanied the changing seasons and times of day. Wherever the traffic was opposed, congested, or even massively disrupted by foreign invaders, the best intervention was with a needle, which could remove the invaders, replenish the supply of *qi*, and drain off surplus or indeed dissolve the congestion. Sometimes it was helpful to burn balls of dried herbs or to do gymnastic breathing exercises, or to administer foods with qualities that were known to exert particular effects on the body.

This new medicine augured a lifestyle that, if faithfully followed, would preclude all kinds of disease, so that the administration of those impressively well-developed pharmaceutical preparations would not be necessary at all. However, the *Huang Di nei jing su wen* mentions many, more or less unpleasant ailments, from diarrhea through diseases of civilization such as back pain to malaria;

from madness through a "prostate illness" with difficulty urinating to the familiar cough, for all of which the adherents of the new medicine looked for words of good advice. And these were copiously dispensed—always in terms of needles, cauterizing, and dietary measures—and excluded pharmaceutical remedies almost entirely. These were considered (expressed in today's terminology) politically incorrect, as explained below.

The individual organs were identified strictly according to their morphology. In one of the ancient texts, the *Classic of Difficult Issues, Nan jing*, there are detailed descriptions of the lungs, heart, spleen, liver, kidneys, small and large intestines, bladder, gall bladder, and stomach, complete with their holding capacities, weight, and number of openings. Only the designation of the heart is not always unambiguous; the same term is sometimes used to indicate the stomach. The function of each inner organ always includes one of the body's outer organs. For example, the liver is also responsible for the functioning of the eyes. Eye problems that are not obviously caused by external influences are accordingly ascribed to liver malfunction and are therefore treated internally.

Modern concepts of diseases that are hidden from sight but lead to characteristic external symptoms perceivable by either patients or doctors are found in the ancient medical texts alongside differentiated treatment instructions, which often specify that the "root," the invisible disease, be treated first, before attempting to ameliorate the "branches," or visible symptoms. Several diseases may manifest themselves simultaneously in different parts of the body, independently of one another, so that the combined clinical picture can appear very complicated.

From today's standpoint it is difficult to determine the origins of a concept that may have begun in an attempt to explain the different temperatures of living organisms, rather like the notion of *calor innatus*, or innate warmth, in the European medicine of antiquity. Such is the case with the concept of "three burners," *san jiao* 三焦, in the ancient Chinese texts. Whatever the source, we can be sure that this concept did not originate in China. It appears as an alien element that swiftly and repeatedly acquired multiple new meanings over the centuries, but its original meaning remains obscure. The theme of changing body heat does not appear at all in the earliest Chinese texts.

It is also remarkable that although both blood and *qi* are identified as essential to life, *qi* is allocated a far greater significance in physiology and pathology, and hence also in therapeutics. Acupuncture, for which there is no reliable literary or archaeological evidence before the late second or early first century B.C.E., was a new treatment modality introduced with the new medicine, and was initially mainly employed as a method of bloodletting. Excess blood was removed from the organism, along with the pathogenic factors that were thought to be located in it, by making openings in the vessels with pointed stones or spikes. Discernable efforts were also made to influence the *qi* by puncturing or applying heat to the outside of the body. Not until near the end of China's imperial age, approximately in the seventeenth century, did acupuncture change into a generally bloodless procedure—a development that nonetheless failed to prevent the rejection of this invasive form of therapy by Chinese social elites. The gentler *tui na* (push-and-pull) massage therapy is attested since the end of the sixteenth century and increasingly took the place of needle therapy among these elites.

The blood played no role in the explanations of healthy and unhealthy lifestyles or in the interpretations of the environmental factors that favored health or disease. *Qi* alone was the essential variable. Every single organ possessed a primordial measure of healthy *qi*. Simultaneously, the *qi* of the various organs, especially of the stomach, circulated in the paired channel systems of the left and right sides of the body. At different, specified places on the body, the flow of *qi* can be detected. The author of the *Nan jing* was the first to make the case that all the *qi* flows in the organism came together at the wrist joint and could be investigated there in order to generate diagnoses.

There is no evidence of any discussion of where, exactly, the blood and the *qi* were supposed to flow, or even agreement among the authors about what the received opinion on this question might be. Several authors saw blood and *qi* flowing either together or separately in the same channels; others suggested that they occupied separate pathways. The details seem not to have been of much interest, and therefore not discussed. At least one author questioned the fact that organs such as the brain did not appear in either the four-six-twelve count of the organs according to the yin-yang theory or the fivefold count according to the Five Phases theory, and were thus excluded from the intellectual edifice of the new medicine. The internal cohesion of these systems left no space for such additional organs.

The power invested in the numerology of the yin-yang and the Five Phases theories determined not only the choice of theoretically acceptable organs but also the classification of diseases. The idea that coughing came from the lungs and was correlated with having a cold clearly reflected earlier opinions. Once the Five Phases theory had been accepted, the idea that only one organ was responsible was no longer meaningful. The new assignment for the medical theorizers was to demonstrate a model wherein the lungs remained the starting point and the cold remained the primary cause, but that also incorporated the other four long-term storage organs (*zang*).

According to this new model, humans are repeatedly exposed to the cold in the course of the five seasons of spring, summer, late summer, autumn, and winter. If, because of internal inadequacies, the body is open to intrusion, then the cold invades the liver in the spring, the heart in summer, the spleen in late summer, the lungs in autumn, and the kidneys in winter. There are direct channels between the liver, heart, spleen, and kidneys and the lungs. Thus the cold can flow through these channels from any of the four other organs into the lungs. This has no consequences, unless the person in question also eats or drinks something cold. This extra cold arrives first in the stomach, which is directly connected to the lungs.

When cold flows from another long-term storage organ into the lungs, or during the autumn flows directly from the cold air into the lungs, and combines there with a second cold current originating from the stomach, the collision of the two sources of cold results in a cough that emerges, as expected, from the lungs. Similarly, as described in chapter 35 of the *Su wen*, there is not just one kind of intermittent fever. Each organ, long-term storage organ and temporary storage organ, has its own variant of intermittent fever, or rather, as the detailed symptom descriptions suggest, malaria.

The intellectual pinnacle in the application of yin-yang and Five Phases teachings to human physiology and pathology is undoubtedly found in the theory of five periods and six *qi*, *wu yun liu qi* 五運六氣. At the basic level, all theorizing had as its cultural goal the demonstration of natural laws that would include all the phenomena in the universe. And it was true that the passing of the seasons was stably predictable in China, as were the times of day. The regularity of ocean tides, for example, could also be taken as a recurring confirmation of the all-encompassing natural cycle of becoming, maturing, life, and death, in accordance with yin-yang and Five Phases teachings. However, the weather, with its climate swings and unpredictably catastrophic droughts and floods, presented a serious challenge to the conviction of an eternal and above all, predictable natural order.

The theory of five periods and six *qi* provided a remedy for this. Using an extremely complicated set of calculations based on completely new understandings of the relationships between the Five

Phases, it now seemed possible to predict the daily climate for up to sixty years in advance. The goal was twofold: the implicit demonstration that everything behaved according to natural laws and the explicit transmission of the idea that one's own health and the desire for autonomy were both best served by aligning oneself with the predictable vagaries of the climate.

8

DEFICIENCIES IN THE CREDIBILITY
OF THE NEW MEDICINE

One of the authors of the *Yellow Emperor's Inner Classic,* "Plain Questions" (*Huang Di nei jing su wen*), advises in chapter 13, "Discard the old and choose the new, and thereby become a true man!" As so often in this text, the passage leading up to the exclamation indicates the parallels between the arts of healing, referring to the human organism, and politics, referring to the management of a state. "Discard the old, choose the new, and thereby become a true man" was not only the message of the authors of the *Huang Di nei jing su wen* (hereafter simply *Su wen*) but also the message of the other text compilations of the later Han dynasty.

These texts are recognized today as the sources of a specifically Chinese medicine and as the distant, but still relevant theoretical underpinnings of today's Traditional Chinese Medicine. Admittedly, when this completely new ideology was first expressed in these texts in an attempt to win over the educated class, it met with little success. Hence the challenge, "Discard the old, choose the new, and thereby become a true man!" The "true man" is the liberated man, the man who holds his fate, *ming* 命, in his own hands, knowing that he must align himself with the laws of nature alone. There was no longer any need to prostrate oneself to the ancestors, demons, or gods.

Perhaps this message, like that of the recent changes in Greek medicine, was part of a larger aspiration for liberation from the rule of kings and emperors. The fact remains that for the overwhelming majority of the literati of the time, the new medicine was not convincing. The numbers of those prepared to "Discard the old and choose the new" must have remained very few. In contrast to the authors of texts of the competing social movements and ideologies such as Confucianism, Daoism, Legalism, and Mohism, whose names are known to us, the authors of the comprehensive and ambitious *Su wen, Ling shu,* and *Nan jing* were lost to posterity.

It is remarkable that in the vast majority of the extant texts, the Yellow Emperor is portrayed not as wise author and creator of medicine but rather as a naïve questioner who is tutored by someone called Qi Bo, a name unknown from other sources. Why, then, is the Yellow Emperor named as the text's author? Can it be that the editors of these compilations remained deliberately anonymous, knowing that they were uttering unmistakable blasphemy on many levels? In none of the ancient bibliographies can we find any named author identified with the texts of the *Ling shu* and *Nan jing.*

Even records of the textual transmission of these books are extremely sparse over the following centuries, among otherwise extremely meticulous lists of texts. For example, the approximately 30,000-character-long doctrine on the five periods and six *qi,* which can be unequivocally dated from its rhyme structure to the Han period, is not mentioned at all in any of the bibliographies. Not until the Tang dynasty, about six hundred years later, did physician-author Wang Bing rescue it from obscurity and incorporate it into the text of the *Su wen.*

The eighth-century author Yang Shangshan, who extracted material from both the *Su wen* and the *Ling shu* and compiled it into a single new text, the *Huang di nei jing tai su,* faded into complete obscurity in China. Perhaps the fact that he was careless enough to assert that even the heart could be infested with evil *qi* had something to do with this: such a view was political blasphemy. The heart in the human organism was the equivalent of the ruler in the political structure, after all. Up until that point, the accepted view was that the actual heart could never be attacked directly by evil influences: it was protected by the "heart envelope." The title of the Chinese emperor, Huang Di, literally translated, means "enlightened god-king" [or: thearch]. To suggest that even the enlightened god-king might be overcome by evil influences represented a radical break with orthodoxy. It is only through an accident of history that the text still exists today. A manuscript copy of it was taken to Japan in the medieval period, where copies were made and deposited in various temple libraries. In China, by contrast, Yang Shangshan's work clearly excited no lasting interest.

The Chinese naturalists who chose not to accept the teachings of the new medicine did not create a unified counternarrative. They were, however, united in their conviction that both demons and the spirits of ancestors existed in the underworld, as well as deities in heaven, and that all of these could exert their influence on human existence, including health and disease. The desire for existential autonomy found no affirmation here. However, one thing was agreed on by both these believers in existential heteronomy,[1] who saw themselves at the mercy of supernatural powers, and the evangelists of the new, secular natural philosophy: life is an eternal battle. Human existence is under constant threat from its enemies.

9

THE ALTERNATIVE MODEL

The View from Illness

For the early Daoists, who embodied the most sustained resistance to the new medicine, evil spirits of the underworld represented eternal threats to the living. Since time immemorial, shamans had plied their trade everywhere. They claimed to be able to communicate with the spirits and win them over for the benefit of a patient's health. These local cults were opposed now by a completely new interpretation that, while it continued to support the idea of the existence of demons from the afterlife, strongly opposed the notion that these evil forces could be deployed for the benefit of humans. The early Daoists maintained that the demons of the underworld were only capable of inflicting harm. To effect a recovery from disease, one had to win over the assistance of deities from the pantheon of heaven.[1]

They were convinced, therefore, of the existence of three worlds, each with its own bureaucratic administration: heaven, earth, and the underworld. Humans must negotiate with the gods in heaven against the forces of the underworld, and for this purpose, the educated and literate priests of Daoism assisted. It was better to entrust oneself to them than to the wildly gesticulating, unrestrained shamans of the local cults. This opinion is reflected in the fact that, toward the end of the Zhou dynasty or around the beginning of the Han, it became necessary to create a new written character to represent the concept of "deceiving" or "to swindle." Accordingly, the responsible literati put two older characters together: to speak, *yan* 言, and dancer/shaman, *wu* 巫, thereby creating the suggestive character *wu* 誣, which is still in use today with the meaning of "to give false evidence/bear false witness."

The task was to convince people that it was not possible to engage the evil spirits of the underworld as allies against disease; instead they were always enemies to be fought against. The priests offered their services, bringing their knowledge of the *Dao*, the correct Way, to help people avoid contracting disease and guide them back to health. They claimed to be familiar with the bureaucracy of heaven and able to summon its assistance for the battle against evil spirits.

Of course, just like allies on earth, heavenly forces did not lend their assistance for nothing. They had to be convinced with offerings to intervene. Thus bribery on earth found its counterpart in heaven. At the same time, sufferers were required to confess their sins and spend some time in isolation in a so-called quiet room in order to reflect on their lives; lastly, they were allowed to return to their normal lives cleansed by repentance. Their transgressions had to be reported to various deities; then priests wrote out amulets that were burned to ashes and dissolved in liquid for the sick person to consume, in order to persuade the deities to intervene against the evil spirits of the dead.

Even though this method of healing involved a very different understanding of the causes of disease and appropriate therapy than the new medicine, its projection of earthly conditions and experiences onto the supposed conditions of heaven and the underworld is just as understandable as the new medicine's projections of political realities onto the inner structures of the human body.

Each of them offered the promise of survival in a universe characterized by violence. In medicine, the "allies" to rely on were the newly described natural laws. Those who were not yet ready to free themselves from the awareness of existential uncertainty relied instead on assistance from deities.

The new medicine was driven by the conviction that understanding and adhering to the secular laws of nature would prevent all occurrences of disease. Acupuncture and dietary modifications were conceived of as therapies for the treatment of small changes in sensitivity rather than of fully developed diseases. However, pharmacy started out from a different set of assumptions, namely that illness was unavoidable and humans must make use of the gifts of nature in order to treat these illnesses. Practitioners of the new medicine distanced themselves as far as possible from the use of the medications so colorfully described in the Mawangdui manuscripts of the early second century B.C.E. In the texts of the *Su wen, Ling shu,* and *Nan jing* we find only occasional mentions of any medications. Around the year 200 C.E., an author called Zhang Ji (styled Zhongjing) wrote a book of formulae in which he applied yin-yang theory to explain the effects of natural drug substances on the human body. But the time was still not right for this kind of bridge building between medicine and pharmacy. His book became known to only a few people, and it was not until the Song dynasty, almost a thousand years later, that it was rediscovered and appreciated, finally achieving widespread acclaim.

During the Tang dynasty, the doctor Sun Simiao (581–682?) quoted from a saying attributed to Laozi, the founder of Daoism, in one of his recipe books: "The fact that I must suffer is a consequence of having a body. Had I no body, what could be the cause of suffering then?"[2] The moment people are born, they become material beings. Matter decays, and no moral behavior, however well intentioned, can prevent this. Sun Simiao followed his quotation of Laozi with this commentary: "So form and matter by themselves will lead to illness.... Only formlessness is free of suffering. If even the wisest are unable to free themselves of suffering, how much less the candles in the wind?"[3]

The early Daoists did not see the sense of the supposed natural laws of yin, yang, and the Five Phases; they also did not see the point of such large political units as a unified China with requirements for writing, laws, long-distance transportation, military power, and an administrative bureaucracy. They rejected the entire structural environment that the new medicine depended on for its principles and justification. In the words of Laozi, documented in chapter 80 of the classic of Daoism, the *Dao de jing*, we see the political alternative clearly described:

> Given a small country with few inhabitants, he could bring it about that though there should be contrivances requiring ten times, a hundred times less labour, they would not use them. He could bring it about that the people would be ready to lay down their lives and lay them down again in defence of their homes, rather than emigrate. There might still be boats and carriage, but no one would go in them; there might still be weapons of war but no one would drill with them. He could bring it about that "the people should have no use for any form of writing save knotted ropes, should be contented with their food, pleased with their clothing, satisfied with their homes, and take pleasure in their rustic tasks. The next place might be so near at hand that one could hear the cocks crowing in it, the dogs barking; but the people would grow old and die without ever having been there. (Arthur Waley translation)

Where there are no laws enforced, people respond to problems in a flexible way. Illnesses are unavoidable, and when necessary, must be treated. The continuation of the pharmacy of the earlier period belonged to this ideological environment, not to the realm of the new medicine, and certainly was not based on the secular natural laws of yin, yang, and the Five Phases. Zhang Ji, who was trying to build a bridge between the two fields, was an outsider and failed to attract followers. For a thousand years, an almost insurmountable ideological rift existed between the medical literature, with its emphasis on needle therapy according to principles of relational theories on one side, and the pharmaceutical literature with its knowledge of drug actions derived from empirical experience, on the other. The medical literature also failed to incorporate the knowledge of the causation of disease by tiny creatures and demons that had been documented in the Mawangdui manuscripts of the second century B.C.E. No procedure imaginable could keep these pathogens away from the body or expel them, should an infestation occur. So they were simply not mentioned in the new medicine. By contrast, in the pharmaceutical literature they continued to be recognized as possible pests to protect oneself against. Yet in this literature we find no hint of the yin-yang or Five Phases theories of systematic correspondence.

Medicinal drugs were objectively described using language that is easily understandable today, with statements that are still valid. We will demonstrate this with four examples. In the Han-era herbal *Shen nong ben cao jing,* the entry on croton seeds, *ba dou* 巴豆, gives descriptions of the same drastic purgative effects that are also given in the historical herbals of Europe. The consciousness-altering powers of the may apple, *lang dang* 莨菪, were also described several hundred years ago in Europe. There was no recorded indigenous lore about the supposed psychotropic applications of ginseng, *ren shen* 人參, in Europe, as this root grew only in East Asia. On the other hand, the dermatological effects of preparations of mercury, *shui yin* 水銀, were well known in Europe.

Ba dou. Flavor: sour; warm. Controls: harm caused by cold, warmth, malaria, alternating sensations of cold and heat. Breaks up concretion and conglomeration illnesses, nodular collections, and hard accumulations, abiding rheum, phlegm aggregation illness, and enlarged stomachs because of water swelling. Cleans out the five long-term storage organs and the six short-term repositories. Clears the pathways of water and grains. Removes rotting flesh/meat. Expels demonic poisons, *gu* attachment illness, and other evil things. Kills worms/bugs and fish. Another name for it is ba pepper.

Lang dang. Flavor: bitter; cold. Controls: toothache. Dislodges worms/bugs, treats flesh blockage and cramps. Facilitates a strong gait and causes people to see demons. Large doses cause one to run wildly about. Taken over long periods, it makes the body lighter, so that one can run as fast as a galloping horse.

Ren shen. Flavor: sweet, slightly cold. Controls: replenishing the five long-term depots. Calms the essence. Strengthens the *hun* and *po* souls. Cures fear and anxiety. Eliminates evil *qi*. Makes the eyes clear. Opens the heart and augments wisdom. Taken over long periods, it makes the body lighter and increases longevity.

Shui yin. Flavor: sour; cold. Controls: *jie* illness and fistula, crust ulcers, white baldness. Kills insects and parasites in the skin. Causes early miscarriages. Clears heat. An antidote to poisoning from gold, silver, copper, and tin. Melting procedures can change it to cinnabar. Taken over long periods, it turns people into immortal hermits.

Recognizable in many of these drug descriptions is the desire to achieve longevity or even immortality through their consumption, either in their natural form or as chemical products. These considerations may represent the origins of alchemy, which came later to the attention of the European educated classes through the mediation of Arabic scholars. Of course, the priority of the traditional Chinese pharmaceutical works was to find and use effective substances and combinations of substances to treat acute illnesses. There was, therefore, a contrast between the focus of the new medicine, which was its promise of safeguarding health, and the traditional pharmacy's primary concern with the treatment of the already sick.

10

RADICAL HEALING

Life as a Form of Disease

When Sun Simiao quoted the saying attributed to Laozi and added his commentary, that "Form and matter by themselves will lead to illness," he was surely already aware of the teachings that came to China with the spread of Buddhism and can be regarded as the most radical form of healing in history. All attempts by means of drugs and other therapies to protect the material substrates of existence against the constant threat of decay were considered merely superficial cosmetics in Buddhism. Birth, aging, death, separation from loved ones, frustration of desires, and other sufferings are all constitutive of the human condition. People attempt to avoid pain and seek out various ways and means to reduce or even eliminate their bodily sufferings. But Buddhism taught that these could offer no true healing. True healing, which is the state of nirvana (in Chinese: *wu bing*, 無病, "free of disease"), can only be reached by achieving the state of nonbeing. There is no way to describe this state.

Within secular European worldviews, death—the end of the lifespan of every single person—is indistinguishable from entering the state of nirvana. But Buddhist doctrine saw it differently. Originating as it did in a period of supposedly universal oppression and suffering, the Indian doctrine offered an avenue of escape, though not without extracting a high price. The European secular world-view provides everyone with the option of an instant way out and transition to nothingness in the form of suicide. Buddhism fore-closed this self-determination of the end of existence by ruling out suicide as a means of shortening the way to nirvana. In Buddhism, existential autonomy does not mean that one frees oneself from the whims of one or more gods or other numinous beings, but that one follows the absolute law, *fa* 法, that undergirds all of existence. This law distinguishes good from evil, and only those who have ac-cumulated a sufficient measure of goodness may be rewarded with admission to nirvana. Thus Buddhism creates an imaginary thresh-old with the easily recognizable goal of establishing some degree of order in the unloved phase of man's earthly existence, and with it, a measure of peaceableness and compassion. The fact that such an ideology succeeded speaks to the horrific conditions of the time. The allure of the possibility of escape from such a potentially end-less cycle of birth, death, and reincarnation into a life full of such suffering was clearly so promising that not a few people were pre pared to commit themselves to the strict requirements of the Bud-dhist moral teachings. As we have seen, the new medicine of the Han era focused on the fear of bodily and perhaps also spiritual suf-fering, in order to encourage particular forms of behavior. The natu-ral law that required such behavior promised existential autonomy to all who assimilated themselves into its secular, relational cos-mology. Buddhism also turned away from existential uncertainty by invoking the personal authority of the individual, but it de-manded a lifestyle that required people to subordinate themselves to a universal law. Living in such a way that the goal of escape from suffering through nirvana could be reached was incomparably more difficult. At the same time that its followers were promised existential autonomy, it was made clear to them that the condi-tions were almost impossible to satisfy. The cold objectivity of the message that "My fate lies in my own hands, not in the authority of Heaven" was accompanied in Buddhism by the sentiment "It's your own fault if you can't make it!"

The principles that the Buddha taught are easily understood: do no evil, do good, and purify your spirit. The meaning of the concept of evil (xie 邪) is a central element in the medicine of the Han era and its underlying moral philosophy. Evil is anything that leaves its proper place and intrudes anywhere it doesn't belong. In Indian philosophy, evil was every act that harmed oneself, another, or both self and other at the same time. To belong to a community that set itself these aspirations was comforting in a time when many people had the impression that reality presented diametrically opposing values. In this philosophy, every deed, every act produced an effect (karma) that would result in appropriate measures of happiness or suffering in a later existence.

Buddha is the physician who heals humanity of the "disease" of existence. His teachings follow the structure of a medical case history. He diagnoses the suffering and identifies its cause. He defines the goal, namely relief from suffering, and shows the patients how to get there. The starting point is the doctrine of the Four Noble Truths, as preached in the Buddha's first sermon. First, life is suffering. Second, this suffering has a cause: the longing for life and the desire for sensual pleasures. Third, there is a way to end this suffering. Fourth, the way to end this suffering is to follow the Eightfold Path. To follow the Eightfold Path, followers must align themselves with: right view, right intention, right speech, right action, right livelihood, right effort, right mindfulness, and right concentration.

Just as the new medicine had defined the opposition between evil (xie 邪) and upright (zheng 正) for its own purposes, Buddhism also described an antagonism between evil (xie) and upright (zheng), while investing them with different meanings. Some of the requirements of the Eightfold Path, such as right view, right intention, and right meditation, require a complex theological definition. Others resemble the Ten Commandments, as for example the third element of the Path, "right speech," which is defined as the avoidance of false or vain speech and comes before the fourth element, "right action," which includes such injunctions as not to kill, not to steal, and to practice chastity. Finally, "right mindfulness" (sometimes translated "right memory") is noteworthy. This requires people to only remember the good and forget the bad. This requirement is perhaps also a result of the situation at the time, when so many bad impressions had been seared into people's consciousness.

We will not go further into the details of Buddhist moral philosophy: that could easily fill several volumes. In the beginning, the Indian teachings were so strictly prescribed that they seemed only accessible to those prepared to tread the arduous path of the self-denying ascetic in order to achieve enlightenment. Much greater numbers of new believers committed themselves later to a less forbidding version: Mahayana Buddhism. Literally translated, Mahayana means "the great vessel" in which everyone can find their place. The cold isolation of the initial doctrine of complete personal responsibility, and the hopelessness it created in those who found themselves incapable of following the arduous Path, was counterbalanced with the new concept of the bodhisattva. A bodhisattva is someone who has carried out so many good deeds in their past lives that they have accumulated immeasurable quantities of good karma, but who chooses not to take advantage of this wealth to achieve nirvana. Instead, they remain available on earth and stand ready to assist less fortunate beings.

The most important bodhisattva for the purposes of medicine and healing was Avalokiteshvara, who has been known in China since the seventh century, in female form, as Guanyin. She represents a source of both warmth and empathy. Guanyin has a thousand eyes, in order to seek the needy everywhere, and she has a thousand arms and hands, in order to assist them. Not unlike the figure of Mary, Mother of God in the Roman Catholic Church, Guanyin is the one to turn to with requests for protection from disease, demons, fire, and water. Because of her willingness to help women suffering under the tremendous pressure to bear a son and to help childless women in need, Guanyin became one of the few numinous beings from whom one might expect compassion.

Buddhism appeared in China with the aspiration to achieve complete freedom from suffering. This is in contrast to Christianity, for example, which still today rejects such freedom from suffering as something unfit for human beings and accordingly restricts human efforts to relieve suffering within narrow, theologically defined boundaries. Buddhism's approach to healing did not entail disallowing any particular therapeutic goals or rejecting any specific forms of therapy as heterodox or inconsistent with its teachings.

Buddhism accepted a uniquely eclectic approach to therapy. As a result, both the secular natural-philosophical theories of the Four Elements (earth, air, fire, and water) from the eastern Mediterranean and the Three Dosas (wind, mucus, and bile) from India were transmitted via Buddhism to China. Neither the Four Elements theory nor its analytical premises was picked up by more than a handful of medical authors from their descriptions in the texts of the Buddhist scriptures. Similarly, the Three Dosas theory stalled because of inadequate translations of its core concepts into Chinese. Without further explanation, the translated versions were simply incomprehensible.

Toward the end of the sixth century, the Buddhist umbrella had finally assembled a form of healing art that recognized six potential causes of disease. This was a mixture of secular and religious causes, which included an unbalanced nutritional status, an imbalance among the Four Elements, excessive meditation, demons and evil deities, and also misconduct in an earlier life. The texts gave the appropriate therapies for each of these different causes, from drug and dietary measures through improved ascetic and meditation practices and regulation of inhalation and exhalation, to the use of exorcistic techniques such as amulets and spells, and finally to introspection, confession, repentance, and penances. Thus it is not possible to make a clear distinction between Buddhist therapies for bodily and spiritual suffering and the other healing practices that existed in China. Especially in the use of drugs and the practices of exorcism we can discern obvious overlaps with Daoist healing methods.

11

BETWEEN ANTIQUITY AND
THE MODERN AGE

None of the theoretical approaches to therapy described in the foregoing chapters was able to marginalize the others and achieve the status of something that we can, in retrospect, identify as "Chinese medicine." We should also bear in mind that, by all indications, the theoretical approaches of the new secular medicine were assimilated by only a very small percentage of the formally educated elites, who were thereby in a favorable position to transmit their reactions to illness. For the period right up until the eighteenth and nineteenth centuries it is scarcely known how the broad masses of Chinese responded to bodily and spiritual afflictions, or how they attempted to prevent them. Research into the history of Chinese medicine over the past few decades has simply analyzed the literary testimony of the elites, and by designating the contents of these texts as "[traditional] Chinese medicine" has led to widespread but equally misleading statements of the kind that start with "The Chinese did such-and-such. . . ."

One thing that can be concluded from the rich literary testimony left by proponents of different therapeutic approaches is that a multitude of individual interpretations developed, especially after the thirteenth and fourteenth centuries, all drawing on the foundation of the medical ideas conceived between about 200 B.C.E. and 300 C.E. For the time being, we will overlook the Buddhist and Daoist explanations for illness. Even though their ideas and practices played significant roles in the attempts of the entire Chinese population to prevent illness and to treat diseases, their religious ideas, particularly the use of exorcistic rituals in therapy, meant that by the time of the twentieth-century efforts to create a respectable "Traditional Chinese Medicine" of the future out of so many heterogenous elements, they were omitted from consideration.

The secular reactions to disease that drew on the ancient texts are certainly impressive in their numbers and diversity. If one considers the entire history of Chinese medical ideas of the past two thousand years, it soon becomes clear that there were three general phases of creativity in which the dynamics of theoretical change led in a new direction. The first of these, already described in previous chapters, occurred during the centuries immediately before, during, and after the Han dynasty, from about the third century B.C.E. until the third century C.E. The next creative phase began around the twelfth century and lasted until the fifteenth century. The third phase began in the late nineteenth century and is ongoing.

When we look back at the history of Chinese and European medicine, it is clear that the creation of medical theories has no innate driving force. There are no historical examples of people introducing fundamentally new theories purely on the basis of their own observations of healthy or sick bodies. Since the beginning of time, all fundamental theories of health and disease have been projections onto the human body of specific fears or confidence in the context of a larger, all-encompassing world order.[1] In the history of both Chinese and European medicine we have seen, time after time, the appearance of new fears and consequently new assurances about who or what could reestablish order. Invariably and subconsciously, medical theorists take up these challenges and respond with new ideas about the nature of health and disease, along with instructions about how to sustain the former and prevent or cure the latter.[2]

In China this led, for example, to the fact that no new medical ideas were taken up during the Tang dynasty (618–906) at all. This might seem a startling claim at first, as China was extremely culturally diverse in this era, with more languages spoken on the streets of the major cities and more visitors and residents from different lands than ever before or since. But it was also a time when no fundamentally new anxieties or convictions appeared to plague its people. Only a very few were haunted by frightening visions of the increasing insignificance of Confucianism in comparison with the competing ideologies of Daoism and Buddhism. These intellectuals and political theorists suggested innovations that would be taken up later, in the Song, Jin, and Yuan dynasties, when China's entire civilization was undergoing major changes.

Bridge Building and Pharmacology

The efforts of the Confucian philosophers of the Song dynasty (960–1279) to present a viable alternative to the growing influence of Daoism and Buddhism were accompanied by a simultaneous and fundamental reworking of medical theory. For more than a millennium, the two traditions of medicine had been clearly divided. The medicine of systematic correspondence, on the one side, appealed through its conformity to natural laws that coincided with demands from Confucianism and Legalism to obey their moral and legal laws. On the other side, the pharmaceutical approach to therapy was more closely aligned with Daoism. This divide was now to be bridged.

The result was a pharmacology of systematic correspondence: an attempt to explain the effects of drugs on the human body in terms of the theories of yin-yang and the Five Phases, and to prescribe accordingly. If the aim had been to create a doctrine that would be adopted by all, or even just a majority of practitioners of Chinese medicine and pharmacy, it was unsuccessful. For the system to work, individual substances had first to be categorized according to yin or yang and the appropriate phase, yet these categories were far from clear. If one theorist designated a substance as sweet, others found it bitter; a substance identified as "cooling" by one person would be considered "cold" or "warm" by others. It proved impossible to achieve a consensus among the different schools of thought.

In addition, several different doctrines arose concerning the fundamental causes of disease. Members of one current considered the main cause of disease to be inadequate care of the stomach and spleen; this was understandable, since the originator of this theory came from a region plagued by lengthy periods of famine and civil war. Others, however, considered too much heat, or alternatively, too much cold as the main cause of disease and oriented their therapeutic interventions accordingly.

The antagonism between these different schools was bitter. As late as the 1930s–'40s, a doctor from North China found this out to his cost. He had had great success healing patients with prescriptions containing Chinese aconite, a substance that was universally recognized as very "hot" or heating. When this physician moved his practice to the "hot" environment of Shanghai and continued to prescribe his "hot" drugs, he drew the ire of all his local colleagues. Even the fact that he was able to save the son of a well-known local physician with his "hot" therapies after everyone else had given up on the case failed to weaken the opposition to his method. After his death, one of his students, who was also the brother of the youth he had saved, published a book about his teacher, who was by then known as "Mr. Aconite." The Shanghai medical community bought up the entire print run and, in 1951, had all the books destroyed.[3]

Handwritten Documentation

For countless authors, it was beyond their financial means to go beyond writing down their views of things to having their writings printed and published. This financial constraint is one reason that using just the printed medical literature gives us the perspective of only one particular section of the educated elite: those who had received a formal education and were wealthy. Only recently have we been able to correct this a little: in 2006 the Berlin State Library and the Ethnological Museum of Berlin acquired a collection of about 1,000 medical manuscripts from the previous four to five centuries. Although this collection does not go beyond the realm of literate authors, it does include a far larger constituency than is represented by the printed literature of medicine.[4]

Among the handwritten books in this collection are some that clearly remained unprinted owing to lack of funds. There are also many family texts and records of simple lay healers and pharmacists whose writings would never have been considered worth printing and publication but are nonetheless revealing and informative. Among them are records of techniques that had not appeared in the printed literature since the Tang dynasty, such as the use of burning lamp wicks to cauterize the skin at acupuncture points or the multitude of formulas for ending a pregnancy with drugs or by mechanical means. For moral reasons, these formulas do not appear anywhere in the printed literature even though they were clearly a frequent necessity. There are also tips for doctors on how best to mislead their patients, for example by passing off cheap and common ingredients as rare and expensive drugs by coloring them or using other processing methods.

A further feature of these manuscript records is that they remind us of medical fads that had a powerful but temporary influence on Chinese medicine. One example is the *yangchong* 洋虫, or "foreign insect." This refers to the consumption of whole specimens of the insect *Martianus desmestoides* Chevrolat. The medicinal use of this insect was mentioned first in 1795 in a book titled *Yao xing kao* (Investigation of drug properties), and slightly later in the *Ben cao gang mu shi yi* (Supplements to the compendium of *materia medica*), which was written around 1800 but not published until 1871. For a while during the nineteenth century, countless numbers of people placed their hopes in this animal drug, which was supposed to nourish both yin and yang aspects of human metabolism, regenerate blood, strengthen the muscles and sinews, eliminate evils from the body, and much more. There are more than a hundred formulas featuring the processing of this insect in the manuscripts. Here is an example: "If a man or woman overeats to the point of feeling bloated and obstructed, with the whole body appearing yellow and swollen and the abdomen tight like a drum, then take seven of these insects that have been steeped in wine."[5]

All of these examples are part of historical Chinese medicine, or what is known today as Traditional Chinese Medicine. What were the failings of this medicine during the eighteenth and nineteenth centuries, that led people to such unrealistic hopes for healing and to so much of the population believing in such outlandish remedies to the extent that they were prepared to ingest them?

Another hitherto unknown find comprises the many libretti for musical plays or folk operas intended to explain the effects of pharmaceutically active substances to the population. In these libretti, all of the roles are played by "people" with the names of drugs. Their good and evil characteristics, their interactions with one another, the places they originate from, and how they should be treated: all this information and more is represented most skillfully in the dialogue between the "persons" (or drugs) and must have left a lasting impression on audiences. All the more so because the mixture of broken taboos, humor, and ribald obscenities in the genre was calculated to be riveting.

Drug Therapy

There are three different therapeutic approaches to be found over the centuries of secular medicine. From a purely quantitative standpoint, the available sources give the impression that the main approach was the use of fixed recipe prescriptions (although there are, of course, no exact statistics). Largely uninfluenced by the promise of theories such as the yin-yang theory or Five Phases theory, medical authors through the centuries compiled an ever-increasing number of prescriptions for the treatment of suffering. Such prescriptions might have been reported by someone as having been effective and thus came to be recommended and recorded, or were formulated according to criteria no longer accessible to us today.

By the twelfth century, or at the latest, the thirteenth century, pharmaceutical manufacturers appear in the historical record. They took the prescription formulas and manufactured and marketed them in wholesale quantities. As early as the twelfth century, the authorities took action against the escalating problem of counterfeiting and decreed that manufacturers must mark their products with an identifiable logo or trademark. Thus began marketing strategies that would continue into the early twentieth century. In particular, manufacturers learned the advertising value of a package design that would attract customers and create brand loyalty, as one says in the business jargon of today. They introduced marketing innovations such as bulk packaging and dual-use containers. For instance, small expensive vases were used as containers for medicinal powders, with the contents and directions for use described on removable paper labels. Once the medicine was consumed, the purchaser could remove the label and employ the vase for displaying flowers or as an ornament.[6] So when the Chinese encountered the emerging European pharmaceutical industry in the nineteenth century, with its prepared remedies and patent formulations, they were not at all surprised.

In contrast, Europeans had no knowledge of Chinese remedies sold as panaceas, promising to successfully treat up to seventy different indications when used in conjunction with specified but ubiquitously available liquids, such as vinegar, wine, rice water, boys' urine, mother's milk, etc., for the individual ailments. It is remarkable that the primary recommended use for these preformulated remedies was for feminine ailments. All these manufactured formulations take no account of the different conditions of individual patients. The focus of treatment was a disease or a particular physical or psychological affliction.

Both the printed and the manuscript collections of remedies contain long lists of all imaginable pains and ailments and recommend treatments for them. The *Ben cao gang mu*, written in the late sixteenth century, contains a total of 11,000 prescription recipes and cites approximately 4,500 different pathological conditions drawn from different texts across the previous centuries.[7] In all of this, there is not a single instruction about making individualized diagnoses based on imbalances of yin or yang, as had been proposed by the pharmacological theory of the Song, Jin, and Yuan eras. The chapters of the *Ben cao gang mu* that do address these theories are in their own separate section and give an impression more of paying lip service than of giving genuine therapeutic advice.

It is difficult to ascertain how many adherents there were of the pharmacological theories of the Song/Jin/Yuan, or how much the theories influenced actual practice. Judging by accounts in the available pharmaceutical literature and from collections of prescriptions, it would appear that the numbers of followers were not particularly significant. The literature on drugs draws on practitioners' knowledge of the individual substances, whether or not they are informed by particular theories. What is impressive about this *materia medica* literature is the dynamic increase in the numbers of substances described over the centuries and in the multiplicity of viewpoints represented.

Starting from the roughly 250 medical substances described in the Mawangdui manuscripts from the second century B.C.E., the number rises in the Han dynasty to 365, the equivalent of the number of days in a solar year, and then to 730 in Tao Hongjing's book of medications from the year 500. The herbals of the Song dynasty, during the twelfth and thirteenth centuries, described more than 1,700 plant, animal, mineral, and man-made items, and Li Shizhen in his *Ben cao gang mu* of 1593 included about 1,900 substances. Authors of individual texts focused on a wide variety of different subfields. There were those that described only those drug plants that could also be used as foodstuffs and those that dealt only with drugs from a specific region. Other writers addressed pharmaceutical methods for processing raw drugs or confined themselves to describing all possible aspects of one particular substance. Only a few drug treatises from the Song/Jin/Yuan period attempted the classification of medicinal substances primarily according to theoretical criteria, but even in these texts we find instructions on how to "Use drugs on the basis of disease symptoms."

Acupuncture and Other Therapies

The significance of acupuncture remained marginal, whether for bloodletting or for regulating a person's flow of *qi*. Acupuncture's fate was tightly bound up with the fate of Confucian ideology, whose values it reflected. There were a few texts on how to conduct acupuncture needling, but markedly fewer than the number of books dealing with drugs and formulas. The best-known acupuncture texts were, first of all, the classic *Jiayi jing* from the third century, and then the great compendium, the *Zhenjiu dacheng*, of 1601. This last text compiled writings from many authors of the past and is still reprinted today.

In the eighteenth century, the government ordered the compilation of all medical knowledge into a single work to be used for teaching purposes; the resulting *Yi zong jin jian* appeared in 1742. This too contained a further review of the achievements of acupuncture. It was clear that it was no longer possible to bring unity to the many divergent schools of thought that had been developing about needle therapeutics, particularly among Qing-era physicians. "Acupuncture" already covered a broad array of different approaches, from those who still believed in the significance of the conduits to those who chose acupuncture points based simply on clinical indications and had no further use for any theoretical paraphernalia.

Taken as a whole, the themes of Chinese medical literature go considerably beyond the narrow confines of the three pillars of therapy mentioned above. Many authors recorded their theoretical insights. Other therapeutic interventions, in the broad sense, included not only the technique known in ancient times as cauterization and today as moxibustion but also the manual therapy known as push-and-pull or *tuina* massage, as well as an elaborate tradition of healthy living similar to its premodern European equivalent, complete with various breathing exercises, physical exercises, and of course, instructions for the preparation and consumption of foodstuffs, among many others.

For inquisitive readers, there were many small, specialized texts as well as large, comprehensive compilations available for consultation. It is therefore understandable that such a rich trove of Chinese medical literature cannot be easily regarded as simply belonging to the past and filed away out of our collective memory. Research into these texts is still in its early stages. In the meantime, progress toward a sober assessment of historical Chinese medicine has been held back by the often defensive and polemical confrontations between those who strive for an independent Chinese medicine and those who would prefer to integrate a few ahistorical fragments into Western medicine.

12

TWO MEDICAL AUTHORS OF THE
MING AND QING DYNASTIES

There are far too few studies of individual physicians from the history of Chinese medicine that might tell us about an individual's ideas or their clinical practices. That is regrettable, for without such fine-grained analyses, the histories we have remain on a mainly abstract or theoretical level, making it easy for us to take individual texts out of context. The personal life of even such a major figure as Sun Simiao (581–682?) remains in shadows, though he is perhaps the most influential clinician in all of Chinese history, and his formularies are regularly reprinted even today. There are biographies of him in the Tang dynasty official histories, along with many anecdotes about him, but little in terms of reliable information, and they convey nothing about Sun Simiao the man, his career, his opinions, or his motivations.[1]

A similar situation holds for the second greatest physician and author in the history of Chinese medicine, Li Shizhen (1518–1593), who was the author and compiler of the great encyclopedia of pharmacy and natural philosophy, the *Bencao gang mu* (published in 1598). In his descriptions of the various medicinal substances are many scattered details about his travels and personal opinions, but there is still no objective and discriminating treatment of his life story in any Western language. [2] By contrast, when we consider the history of European medicine since the Renaissance we find biographies of individual physicians burgeoning in number and rendered in increasing detail as time goes on. The disparity in the numbers of available biographies of Chinese compared with European physicians results in a serious deficit in our ability to make meaningful comparisons between these two medical traditions.

There are, however, a couple of exceptions. Wan Quan (1500–1585?) and Xu Dachun (1693–1771) were both physicians and authors, although if one were to ask Chinese historians of medicine for names of the most outstanding representatives of Chinese medicine from the Ming and Qing eras, neither would be the first to spring to mind. In some ways, this makes their biographies more valuable, as we can infer that, in spite of their undoubted idiosyncrasies, they are also representative of many of the literate elite medical authors of their time.

Wan Quan

Wan Quan was born in 1500, and by his own account, he was the grandson of a skillful pediatrician.[3] We should take this claim with a grain of salt, however. Because there were no public standards by which to measure the quality of a doctor in traditional China, nor even any formal courses of education, much of the credibility of a doctor depended on being the heir to a family tradition of medicine. This is reflected in a saying from one of the ancient classics, often quoted throughout the imperial period: "If a doctor isn't [at least] the third generation, don't take his medicine." This explains why there are often claims to a family tradition of medicine in the self-representation of historical figures and even of Chinese practitioners of TCM in the modern West. The truth content of these statements is frequently unverifiable.

Wan Quan's father, by contrast, is a known historical figure. He migrated from the overpopulated region where he was born to a new area that promised a better livelihood. Once there, he opened a drugstore where he sold the medicinal formulas that had been handed down in his family. To have such family recipes was also not unusual: because professional doctors had a very low social status and their competence was widely mistrusted, every household preserved some basic medical knowledge. This was especially true of so-called "proven remedies" that had shown themselves effective against particular ailments. Calling in a doctor to attend a sick relative was done only as a last resort, when one no longer had confidence in one's own healing abilities.

Wan Quan's father had hoped for a better future for his son, one that did not involve a medical career. Obedient to his father's wishes, the young man devoted himself to preparing for a much more prestigious and advantageous career in the official civil service. However, in spite of achieving excellent marks in the civil service exams, he was denied this route to wealth and power, supposedly as a result of slander spread by other candidates who were resentful of him. If Wan Quan had truly been part of a family tradition of medicine, once he started to practice he would have gradually acquired a local reputation for competence that went beyond simply relying on the family name. His reputation would then have spread beyond his local area. This is not what happened, however. Not until late in his life did Wan Quan begin to experience success.

After he abandoned his ill-fated attempts to become a civil servant, Wan Quan was so poor that he was forced to work as an itinerant healer, a role that was generally despised by the respectable population. In general, such healers traveled from place to place selling just one kind of drug. They could only make their living by dissuading the people they encountered from their initial skepticism and convincing them that this drug was exactly the right one to treat whatever ailment the onlookers were suffering from. The popular saying that "To sell medicines or tell fortunes, all you need is the gift of gab" indicates the kind of occupation it was.

Itinerant healers often possessed handbooks containing hundreds of preformulated scripts that seem quite psychologically sophisticated from today's point of view. These scripts provided the answers to use when encountering skeptical questions, or to help refute derogatory remarks made by the local population, to whom they appeared as untrustworthy strangers. Only when a modicum of trust had been established would someone from the circle of bystanders consent to engage the unknown healer in the kind of dialogue that would facilitate a diagnosis and, eventually, the sale of an appropriate medication.[4] It is likely that Wan Quan was well schooled in these negotiations by his apothecary father.

Ever since the Song dynasty in China, there has been an increasingly close connection between medicine and pharmacy. This is in stark contrast to the situation in Europe, where an initiative of the thirteenth century attempted—even if not entirely successfully—to prohibit physicians from selling drugs, so as to prevent them from using their diagnoses to generate sales. The consequences of this initiative are still with us today. In China, by contrast, it became normal practice for doctors to work as employees of an apothecary's shop, thereby generating extra revenue for their employers. This practice continues today. Various medical recipe books of the Song era encourage their readers not to see a doctor, but to first identify their complaint using the book's symptom lists, then go directly to the apothecary to purchase the appropriate treatment.

Under these circumstances, many doctors had no other choice but to put themselves in the service of an apothecary shop in order to acquire a client base. Still today, the larger drugstores in the People's Republic of China have several doctors on the staff, whereas smaller drugstores might employ a single doctor. In this system there is no incentive to prescribe only a few drugs or even none at all. Furthermore, the distinction between medical and pharmaceutical roles has remained blurred ever since. Many pharmacists could not afford to hire a physician and preferred to diagnose and treat themselves. In modern China it is still possible to find hospitals that entrust the diagnosis and treatment of patients to experts in traditional Chinese pharmacy.

But Wan Quan was no ordinary itinerant healer; his learned status made it possible for him to move beyond this occupation and become the resident physician in his own drugstore, from which he was able to afford several concubines and consequently to bring many children into the world. Medicine could be a very lucrative occupation. It is not unusual to read in the memoirs of Chinese physicians that they were motivated to become doctors only after the medical bills from the treatment of a parent had driven the family to financial ruin. Nian Xiyao (fl. 1725), who had been an official and was also a medical author, expressed just such an apparently widespread sentiment when he said: "Doctors of old practiced on the basis of extensive study, in order to benefit the people. Doctors of today practice without studying at all, in order to enrich their own families."[5]

Today in China, it is not particularly unusual for patients with a life-threatening illness to refuse treatment because they have inadequate health insurance, thereby prematurely ending their lives. The alternative to immediate death is a lengthy course of treatment, very likely also ending in death, and additionally causing financial ruin for the patient's family. The long history of similar circumstances has had the effect of preparing less wealthy members of the population to accept the shortcomings of the current system.

In his own practice, Wan Quan concentrated on pediatrics, and in particular on smallpox, which constituted the greatest threat to children's lives. Not every case of smallpox ended in death, of course, and it is very likely that some patients who were diagnosed with it would, by today's diagnostic criteria, be diagnosed with other illnesses. Regardless of the therapeutic abilities of their doctors, it is highly probable that some proportion of the patients recovered during medical treatment, perhaps because of it, or perhaps even in spite of it. The foundations of Chinese medical therapy built up over the previous two thousand years provided the required prescriptions.

Whatever the reason behind the formulation of a particular prescription, it would be identified as a "tried-and-true recipe" if the patients showed improvement during treatment with it. Such recipes were handed down by word of mouth and collected in private family medical notebooks. Both lay healers and educated physicians collected long lists of reputedly effective prescription recipes, and some businesses even handed them out to their customers as gifts. If someone was looking to improve the balance of their karmic account in preparation for the afterlife, they could always add credit by writing a tried-and-true prescription on a piece of paper and posting it somewhere public, so that passersby would be able to copy it down and thereby pass along the good deed. Occasionally the recipe poster would attempt to ensure this by threatening that "Anyone who fails to pass it on will suffer from the same disease that this prescription is effective against!"

It must be conceded that very few of these prescriptions would have demonstrated the same effectiveness when used a second time, even against apparently identical diseases, leading people to continually devise new prescriptions that were, in turn, added to the canon of received remedies. One can already see the beginnings of this dynamic in the two hundred-plus handwritten recipes discovered in the excavated Mawangdui tombs from the second century B.C.E., a number that had swelled to 5,300 recipes by the time of Sun Simiao's prescription collection in the seventh century C.E. The tradition reached its highest point in the fifteenth century when the prescription collection *Pu ji fang* included a grand total of about 60,000 recipes. By contrast, the famous encyclopedia of pharmacy and natural history of the sixteenth century, the *Ben cao gang mu*, recorded only 11,000 recipes.

The Berlin collection of handwritten Chinese medical books from the last four to five hundred years is evidence of the wide distribution of such private medical recipe collections. Approximately 400 of the 1,000 volumes are recipe collections, with a combined total of more than 45,000 entries. Only some of this great number of recipes are also found in the printed medical literature; clearly many procedures were transmitted without ever reaching the threshold of acknowledgment by publication. Among these are recipes consisting of only a single ingredient, or recipes that relied on constituents only available in a particular local area. However, there are many prescriptions for procuring abortions, and also remedies for treating or reviving patients who have attempted suicide with a variety of different poisons.

Physicians in the Ming dynasty who considered themselves learned could not simply turn to such lists of hundreds of recipes that claimed to have been effective against similar cases once upon a time and conduct their treatments by trying out one after the other until one of them turned out to be successful. Learned doctors counted as learned precisely because of their ability to provide an explanation for their patients' aches and pains, and it was assumed that they constructed their treatment formulas based on these theoretical insights. The pressure to provide this kind of theoretical explanation increased noticeably after the developments of the Song, Jin, and Yuan dynasties.

The newly created pharmacological theories of the time contributed to the goal of being able to connect, at a theoretical level, the observed effects of drugs on the body with explanations of the symptoms of disease.[6] The ability to base their drug recommendations in such pharmacological terms provided doctors with an opportunity to demonstrate their learned status. This was certainly also a reaction to the efforts by the Song dynasty government to make visits to a doctor superfluous by publishing lists of symptoms together with appropriate treatment recipes. Armed with the new theoretical insights, doctors were able to demonstrate that identical symptoms could nonetheless be due to different diseases of the human organism. Someone who didn't recognize these internal differences and treated patients with identical symptoms the exact same way would, according to this new medical rhetoric, bring much misfortune to the sick.

Wan Quan was one of those doctors whose ultimately unsuccessful educational preparation for the Chinese civil service led him to consider himself a learned gentleman, and who relied on the explanatory models of theoretical pharmacology to convince his patients or their families of his competence. Such efforts to convince were unavoidable given the low level of professionalization of doctors accompanied by the high level of mistrust on the part of their clients. If a patient died, it was not unusual for the last doctor to have treated them to be charged with incompetence, fraud, or even murder, in each case with the correspondingly unpleasant consequences. Doctors were forced to protect themselves on all sides so that each of their lucrative therapeutic interventions did not simultaneously present life-threatening risks. The insurance scheme adopted by itinerant doctors was to move on immediately so as to never encounter their patients again after treatment. Resident doctors proceeded differently. They explained their assessment of the client's situation beforehand, seeking their consent to the proposed therapy, and as far as their level of literacy allowed, relied on a more or less detailed written documentation of their procedures.

Some doctors had these case histories printed for use as promotional literature. The familiar story line goes like this: a patient who has failed to respond to domestic treatments or whose case has been mishandled by other doctors finally turns to the author, who succeeds in curing him and explaining the case. Such case records are instructive for several reasons. The reader is led to believe that all the author's treatments were successful. The reader's attention is also repeatedly drawn toward the conclusion that most doctors are incompetent and that great care must be taken in the selection of a good one—and the author turns out to be the only good one available.

European doctors struggled for hundreds of years to successfully persuade public opinion that only a competent insider was qualified to assess the quality of a colleague. In the process of achieving this status of an official profession, public criticism of colleagues was highly undesirable, as it was a continual reminder of lapses of competence within doctors' ranks. The same rationale informed the prohibition against doctors advertising their services, which is still in force in Europe. To the public, these measures were designed to give the impression that all doctors who had completed the required education and passed the necessary exams were equally competent and trustworthy. Only after having established this foundation was it possible for the medical profession in Europe to gain the right to evaluate malpractice cases themselves rather than be judged by lay outsiders. Such a situation could never have emerged in China. A standardized education with final examinations as the basis for a license to practice was never introduced, and doctors never came up with initiatives to demarcate the boundary between themselves and the laity, such as using their own technical terminology. Instead, doctors looked out for their own personal interest and took pains to depict their colleagues as incompetent.[7]

It took Wan Quan at least twenty years to be accepted by the families of the upper classes. Apparently he was already fifty-eight years old by the time a high official engaged him for the first time, to treat his only son. His therapeutic success in this case gave him access to high-class patients from then on. By that time he had already published several books on the subjects of harm caused by cold disorders, pox diseases, general pediatrics, and explanations of and treatments for fertility problems. These writings served the additional purpose of summarizing his knowledge into a systematic form for passing on to his sons and other students. We should emphasize that Wan Quan, like so many of his colleagues of the Ming and Qing, went beyond maintaining the heritage of the medical classics of antiquity and incorporating the theoretical innovations of the Song/Jin/Yuan era: he was also prompted by his own observations to come to new discoveries and interpretations. For example, his advice for successful "health maintenance" (*yangsheng* 养生) was combined with what we could today consider psychological aspects. These had no grounding in the classical theory of Chinese medicine, but many of them seem convincing and compatible with modern ideas.

To summarize and conclude, in Wan Quan's work we see a reflection of the zeitgeist of the late Ming dynasty, which may be regarded as the high point of theoretical complexity in the history of Chinese medicine. The care taken to explain every individual case on its own merits—what today might be called a kind of "personalized medicine"—gave rise to texts that failed to identify a common denominator or common causative agent for conditions such as diarrhea with cramps. Instead an individual therapy might be chosen based on whether the patient bent over in the form of a worm, a dog, a crow, or other animals or objects. This method was in stark contrast to the long tradition of collections of established formulas that continued to be sold by large-scale manufacturers as ready-made medications and marketed irrespective of the age, sex, or other characteristics of the individual patients.

Just two hundred years later, Xu Dachun, another Chinese doctor, gave a very sober analysis of the situation. In his view, Chinese medicine had lost its essential constituents; he described it as a "lost tradition."

Xu Dachun

Xu Dachun was born in 1693 into a family from Wujiang city, Jiangsu province, who could trace their status as officials and literati back as far as the Song dynasty. Xu Dachun's grandfather Xu Qiu (1636–1708) was a landscape artist, poet, and contributor to the official history of the Ming dynasty. His father, Xu Yanghao, had made a name for himself as an expert in irrigation systems. By the time of Xu Dachun's birth, however, the family was impoverished, which may be the reason the young man did not receive the kind of education that would have qualified him to take part in the official civil service examinations. Nonetheless, he became knowledgable in irrigation and river control systems, in continuation of his father's expertise.

Without the benefit of a formal education, he schooled himself in medicine, philosophy, and music, becoming an author of books, essays, and poetry. He achieved the most recognition for his occupation as a doctor and claimed authorship of four medical books. Three of these were commentaries on ancient medical texts: one on the *Nan jing*, the classic work on diagnosis; one on the oldest Chinese pharmaceutical work, the *Shen nong ben cao jing*; and one on Zhang Ji (Zhang Zhongjing)'s *Shang han lun*, the first Chinese text to describe the relationship between the theory of yin and yang and the effects of drugs on the human body. His final work is the highly informative, retrospective *Yi xue yuan liu lun, Treatise on the Origin and Development of Medicine*, written in 1757.[8] In his lifetime, Xu Dachun achieved fame that reached far beyond his immediate circle. In 1771, the then seventy-eight-year-old was summoned to Beijing for a medical consultation with a high official; he died there later that same year.

It is not difficult to detect Xu Dachun's conservative orientation from his writings. In fact, many members of his social class were dissatisfied with the political situation of the time. China was ruled by an alien dynasty, the Manchus, a formerly nomadic people of the northern steppes. In 1644 they had decisively overthrown the previous dynasty, the Ming. Even though the Ming (1368–1644) had been ruled by Han Chinese, its rulers had adopted and continued several of the "foreign" methods of the previous administration, the Yuan (1234–1367), which was another alien dynasty ruled by Mongols. This led many nationalists of Xu Dachun's time to claim that all of the previous five centuries represented a loss of Chinese identity.

Intellectuals who looked for the causes of this regrettable state of affairs first blamed the Neo-Confucian innovations of the Song dynasty for China's decline, but their continuing search for authentic Chineseness in the past led them eventually to the Han dynasty, the first great flourishing of the united empire. Interestingly, these attempts to recover the roots of Chinese culture appeared first in medical theory and were only later manifested in political theory. Xu Dachun's statements show clearly where he placed the blame for China's situation: the problems and weaknesses of the present, he stated repeatedly, were the inevitable consequences of straying from the path of the sages of antiquity. Pragmatic and direct approaches to solving problems—in politics as in medicine—were far more effective than those that relied on excessive and artificial theorizing.

Xu Dachun was scorchingly critical of the theoretical innovations that began during the Song dynasty. He characterized as irrelevant the efforts of physicians of the Song/Jin/Yuan era to explain the effects of drugs on the human body according to the theory of correspondences between yin-yang and the Five Phases. We can assume that Xu Dachun would have considered doctors like Wan Quan less than exemplary: "The streets are filled with the spirits of those who have been killed by such crimes."

Xu's reverence for the "ancients" led him to take them as perfect models for all time, and to hold the *Huang Di nei jing* as the only valid guide to medical practice. He detected questionable deviations from the pure teachings of the *Huang Di nei jing* even in as early a text as the *Nan jing*. In spite of his orientation toward an idealized past, Xu Dachun was not a stubborn, narrow-minded conservative. The *Yi xue yuan liu lun* bears witness to the great intellect, flexibility, and even humor of its author.

In fact, many of Xu Dachun's statements would not appear strange to Western readers, as for example when he emphasized the significance of medicine. In the sayings of the most famous philosopher of the Song dynasty, Zhu Xi (1130–1200), are several statements illustrating the low esteem in which professional healers were held by orthodox Confucians. For example, concerning the renowned physician and author of the Tang dynasty, Sun Simiao, Zhu Xi commented, "He was a well-known scholar of literature. But because he earned his living from medicine, he was relegated to the status of an artisan. How regrettable!"

After Zhu Xi disparaged medicine as a *xiao dao* 小道, or "lesser way," and classified it alongside such grubby occupations as gardener, many Chinese physician-authors felt duty-bound to register their opposition. Xu Dachun's response reads like this: "Humans occupy the most important position on earth, and the fate of humans on earth depends on medicine [or: doctors]."

Even though Zhu Xi had condemned the practice of medicine as an occupation unworthy of a gentleman, Xu Dachun maintained a different view: "If a profession is unworthy, no educated person will want to practice it. The uneducated are, however, incapable of grasping its subtleties."

The question was, what abilities could really be attributed to medicine? Why were individual lifespans so different? Did each person have a (today we might say "genetically") predetermined lifespan? Is it possible to engage in practices to extend one's life— perhaps even indefinitely? Xu Dachun was completely forthright in his opinion on this: "The teachings of 'nurturing life' suggest that by following them, it is possible for anyone to avoid death. Such teachings are nonsense! . . . In the moment we receive life, we also have a predetermined allotment of it."

The evil influences that prevent humans from living out their predetermined lifespans come from people's own self-destructive behavior and from conditions in the natural environment that are detrimental to health. The role of medicine, therefore, is to assist people, as owners of their own health, to take responsibility for not injuring it themselves, and to help them avoid or overcome the damaging effects of changes in the natural environment.

The question of whether the body could heal itself, so that healing from disease might occur with or without therapeutic interventions, was only rarely addressed in Chinese texts. Even though Chinese observers from ancient times had noticed that some illnesses heal by themselves, there is little discussion in Chinese literature about why that might be so, in contrast to the rich European literature on the same topic. Xu Dachun also does not seem to have given much thought to the issue of why some diseases are self-limiting, but he did communicate his observation of the phenomenon:

If a disease does not run a fatal course, the observable symptoms will gradually recede, and the inner injuries will be gradually repaired. It will heal itself. . . . I believe that there are some people who, when they get sick, recover spontaneously without treatment, others who struggle to recover without medical intervention, and yet others who cannot recover without medical help and will die.

The consequence of this observation is that not all diseases need treatment. Often a successful recovery should not be credited to the success of a doctor or to the drugs, but rather to the characteristics of the particular disease. The concept of "powers of self-healing" that was devised in Europe cannot be found in the history of Chinese medicine. Nonetheless, Xu Dachun was critical of the usual obligation to intervene early in every case where a doctor was called in to see a patient.

Two issues that Xu Dachun addresses make it almost seem that he had anticipated some of the twentieth-century Western misconceptions about the unique features of traditional Chinese medicine. These issues concern questions of causality and location of disease. If medicine, as envisioned by Xu Dachun, was to help prevent people from shortening their predetermined lifespans through their own actions, then it had to be capable of identifying the causes of each person's illness. That is, after all, the ultimate meaning of existential autonomy as applied to a medicine based on natural laws. Diseases are not the result of the arbitrary decisions of a supernatural authority figure; rather, they are the comprehensible and therefore generally avoidable consequences of violations of particular laws of nature. Xu Dachun had a clear opinion on this topic too: "Whenever a disease arises, it must have a cause. . . . Whenever a person is suffering, we speak of disease. The reason for the appearance of disease is called its cause."

Identical ailments might be the results of different causes. Xu Dachun aligned himself with the original teachings of the *Huang Di nei jing* in identifying causes: they were the seven emotions as internal causes, and the intrusions of any of the six changing climatological *qi* as external pathogens. Diseases caused internally began in the "long-term depots," *zang*, and "short-term repositories," *fu*, organs. Diseases originating from external causes began in the conduits and network vessels.

Even though Chinese medicine supposedly places so little value on the relationship between morphology/anatomy and pathology, Xu Dachun thought about disease in markedly localized ways. This reminds us that the immediate comprehension of analogous notions introduced to China from Europe only a hundred years later is not in the least surprising. One of Xu Dachun's chapters is titled "Concerning Intra-abdominal Obstruction Illnesses." If Xu Dachun had had the opportunity to meet with his contemporary, the Italian morphologist Giovanni Battista Morgagni (1682–1771), author of the 1761 work *De Sedibus et Causis Morborum* (On the locations and causes of disease), his chapter would have provided the foundation for an interesting exchange of professional expertise.

The detailed contents of Xu Dachun's chapter on "intra-abdominal obstruction illnesses" are not reproduced in any contemporary Western book on Traditional Chinese Medicine. This modern literature is compiled in order to emphasize the contradictions between Western medicine and TCM, and leaves no role for reminders of their common ground. Xu Dachun wrote:

> In cases of liver obstruction illness, a slight pain is discerned in the flanks. After a while, the patient will vomit pus and blood. Obstruction illness in the small intestine is similar to that of the large intestine, except that its location is a little higher. Obstruction illness of the bladder is accompanied by abdominal pains near the upper edge of the pubic hair. Such pains are felt when the skin is touched. Urination becomes painful and difficult.

Xu Dachun also had precise notions about the course of disease. A specific cause resulted in a disease. A disease has a specific initial bodily location. Some diseases remain static in a particular location, while others move around the body: "Some diseases are transmitted and transform themselves according to fixed rules. . . . As soon as the disease transmits, one must [investigate] both primary and secondary locations."

The investigation was oriented according to the signs of disease:

> The general term for an ailment is a "disease," and every single disease necessarily has multiple signs. For example, when the greater yang [conduit] suffers wind damage, then that is the disease. The signs of this disease are the aversion to wind [drafts], fever, spontaneous sweating, and headache that accompany it.

According to this, disease is a theoretically comprehensible construct, to be identified by a physician. The signs of disease constitute the reality perceived by the patients. "Diseases and their signs of suffering appear in innumerable combinations. One must locate the origin and then sort out the end points."

Diagnosis allowed for an exploration of whether a patient was suffering from one or several diseases, due to one or several causes; where the disease was currently located and if transmitting, where it had migrated from; and what kinds of disease signs and symptoms were evident. Finally, it allowed for the determination of primary and secondary signs, or signs of the primary disease and detection of other comorbidities. From there it was possible to design therapy to treat multiple diseases and signs of disease either simultaneously or separately one after the other, or to treat a single disease without regard to the others, or indeed not to treat at all.

These are just a few excerpts from the rich contents of the *Treatise on the Origin and Development of Medicine*. They are sufficient to demonstrate the high clinical standards of the author. His contemporaries, as he often reminds the reader, were rarely up to these standards:

> Doctors of today have completely abandoned the good methods of the sages.

> The chain of transmission of medical knowledge is broken.

> Contemporary doctors don't even know the names of diseases.

> In recent years it seems that people who select doctors and people who practice medicine are both equally ignorant.

> I greatly deplore the fact that since the Tang and Song eras, educated gentlemen have neglected to contribute to the abundance of medical knowledge. Instead, they have designated medicine as an unworthy occupation. This is the cause of great losses in the scholarly medical tradition.

It is impossible to know how many of Xu Dachun's contemporaries shared his opinions. However, he was certainly not the only person to voice such disparaging assessments of the quality of Chinese medical doctors. So when the Chinese reformers and revolutionaries of the early twentieth century, prompted by the perceived inferiority of Chinese culture, science, and above all, medicine when compared with those of the West, uttered their biting critiques of China's historical medical practices, such criticisms had also been made long before the confrontation with Western medicine.

The reputation of doctors of traditional Chinese medicine at the end of the Qing dynasty may also have suffered from the fact that fewer and fewer candidates for the civil service were able to achieve the goal of educated officialdom for which they had prepared, and—like Wan Quan and innumerable others who shared the same fate—contented themselves with the practice of medicine instead. A Christian missionary who observed the situation at first hand described it like this: "The profession of medicine is considered an excellent conduit, or waste pipe, to carry off all the literary bachelors who cannot attain to the superior grades, or pretend to the mandarinate; and China is consequently swarming with doctors."[9]

When Xu Yanzuo (fl. 1895) expressed his opinion of the doctors of his homeland on paper, his words connected with the past and anticipated the critics of the first half of the twentieth century:

It is rare for people to die of their diseases, but many die from the drugs they are prescribed. Those who practice this profession [of medicine] concern themselves first of all with clever rhetoric, and with this, they kill people. The fact that they are able to achieve fame in this way is truly deplorable![10]

II

MODERN AND CONTEMPORARY TIMES

13

THE CONFRONTATION WITH THE
WESTERN WAY OF LIFE

In the fifteenth century, China commanded a naval armada the likes of which was not seen again anywhere in the world until the twentieth century, in terms of both size and manpower. It included 60 so-called "treasure ships," *baochuan* 宝船, with the enormous length of 135 meters and a width of up to 55 meters. Each ship's firepower was assured with 24 bronze cannons. In order to transport and provide logistical supplies to the great warships with their total of 28,000 military (including cavalry with horses), the treasure ships were followed by a flotilla of junks, so that the commander, Admiral Zheng He (1371–1433), presided over more than 300 vessels. Artisans such as blacksmiths and experts in astronomy and navigation were available to deal with all possible problems that might befall such maritime expeditions. Doctors, pharmacists, and cooks tended to the bodily well-being of the crew; Buddhist monks and Muslim clerics were responsible for their spiritual condition.

Zheng He led his armada through the South China Sea seven times, in 1405, 1407, 1409, 1413, 1417, 1421, and 1430. They traveled around today's south Vietnam toward Java, Sumatra, Sri Lanka, and India, and even farther, passing Hormuz in today's Iran and reaching Aden and Mogadishu, finally arriving at the coast of East

Africa somewhere in the region we now call Kenya. Where the opportunity presented itself, they bartered their wares. They brought with them large supplies of porcelain and silk; metalware of silver, bronze, and other metals; and tea and candles. We can assume that these precious items, coming from faraway China, were highly sought after. On the return voyage, the ships brought other desirable luxury goods: pearls and ivory, spices such as cinnamon and pepper, rare woods such as black bamboo, medicinal herbs, and also exotic animals such as elephants, lions, zebras, parrots, and giraffes.

For reasons that are still unclear even today, in the second half of the fifteenth century forces in the Chinese imperial administration succeeded in undermining the value of these expeditions. By the beginning of the sixteenth century, this went as far as a total prohibition on overseas voyages. Not only all the documentation associated with Zheng He's extensive expeditions was ordered to be destroyed, but so were any ships capable of sailing the high seas. The many foreign goods and exotic animals that had been brought into China from faraway places seem to have elicited no great interest or desire to extend trading relations or further imports. From now on, China was to be self-sufficient.

In 1793, at the urging of the British East India Company, King George III (1738–1820) sent a mission to China under the leadership of Lord Macartney. The English were hoping to persuade the court in Peking to open up the huge Chinese empire to trade. Macartney traveled with different kinds of expensive gifts and showcased many attractive examples (or so the English thought) of the productive capabilities of their native land. The Chinese court sent escort ships and other vessels bedecked with banners that clearly read "Embassy from England delivering tribute payments," and received the members of the mission with impressive displays of ceremony. Macartney, as ambassador, was granted a personal audience with the emperor. However, in September of that year the emperor conveyed his rejection of the British suggestions in the form of two edicts.

It took the British another fifty years to find a reason to violently coerce China to open up. The First Opium War represented the first link in a long chain of aggressive acts. The results of the military conflicts on the Chinese side were initially shaming, and then increasingly humiliating as time went on. Each capitulation by the Chinese defenders was followed by peace negotiations, which generally ended in the victors imposing their demands with a diktat. These demands consisted of increasing encroachments on the territorial integrity and political and economic sovereignty of China. After the British beginning came the Second Opium War not long afterward, into which France inserted itself along with Britain. The Netherlands, Portugal, and Spain had already succeeded in acquiring small parcels of land as their colonies; Russia appropriated huge stretches of land in the northeast; the United States successfully asserted the right to enjoy the same rights as the belligerent European powers; and the Germans came to the scene relatively late with their annexation of Qingdao (formerly Tsingtao). Finally, the Japanese showed themselves to be the most avaricious pillagers of all. The "Twenty-One Demands" they presented to the young Republic of China at a time when it was still looking for structural support exceeded all the previous encroachments of the United States and Europe. Japan's behavior was a contributing factor to the demise of the Chinese empire in 1911, in spite of its long and unique, if changing, structural and cultural history.

This, described in the briefest of terms, was the profound rupture in the cultural history of China, leading to a series of changes that were more radical than any previous reforms. It is impossible, using these few words, to convey the depth of the trauma in the collective consciousness that was set off by these searing events, and the ways their aftermath affected both domestic and international politics. China might have—understandably—reacted emotionally, like other regions of the world that perceive themselves to be humiliated by Western culture and military superiority. China might well have indulged in mindless terrorism in order to give vent to its rage, in the continued hope that with its many thousands of years of proud history, it would still end up as the victor. But China went in another direction, following the way of reason. Through an extremely painful process, the collective consciousness settled on an attitude that was willing to learn those things from the West that were unknown in China and thereby acquire the necessary means to catch up with them.[1]

China did not reform itself, however much that word may turn up in the literature. Rather, China underwent a revolution lasting a hundred years and ended up with a situation very different from that at the beginning. At first it seemed that all that would be necessary to destroy the Japanese army at the beginning of the Sino-Japanese War in 1895 was to buy up the arsenal produced by arms manufacturers such as Krupp in Germany, and emulate the way the German army had defeated the French with these same weapons in the war of 1870–1871. This was shown to be an illusion when the Japanese delivered a crushing defeat. Gradually, people came to realize that there was a kind of logistics behind the superior technology of the West, inseparable from many other aspects of Western culture and civilization. The Chinese desire to innovate turned increasingly toward Western culture for inspiration, and reformers and revolutionaries focused their gaze ever more widely, drawing on Western sciences, logic, and of course also modern medicine.

What all this meant for indigenous science was that it came under scrutiny and was dismissed as worthless in almost every sense. Chinese medicine, after two thousand years of being associated with the expectation that it could cure the sicknesses of the Chinese people, now became a symptom and symbol of the sickness of China and its civilization. For everyone who was striving for the well-being and future of the country, the first priority for healing China was now the "healing" of Chinese medicine. At first, many writers thought it was still possible to correct the weaknesses of their indigenous healing art with infusions of Western science. By the beginning of the twentieth century, however, a conviction spread that the ailing China could only be made strong and healthy by replacing Chinese medicine in its entirety with Western medicine.

Regaining health and strength were more than simply metaphors for the necessity of political revitalization in China. The spread of social Darwinist ideas in the context of China's social and political failings was causing some intellectuals to experience premonitions of catastrophe, against which Western medicine seemed to be the only viable possibility for restoring the physical health of the Chinese people so that they might withstand the battle for survival against the West.

Already in 1895, Kang Youwei (1858–1927) had spearheaded the "ten-thousand-word petition" to the emperor, in which he had urged the creation of a modern health care system. In the radical departure from the past that this document proposed, physicians of Western medicine would not only be responsible for the health of the people but also be entrusted with leading all political affairs. This was the context in which the philosopher and journalist Liang Qichao (1873–1929), another of the reformers of this period, founded a Society for Medical Welfare. As he explained, he was induced to take this step because of the grievous state of traditional Chinese medicine. In order to avoid complete extermination, China had to go beyond improving its intellectually inferior situation and pay particular attention to the health and physical strength of its population. For this purpose, only Western medicine was appropriate: "Preserving the people must start from medicine!"[2]

Liang Qichao developed Kang Youwei's ideas in direct opposition to those of Song dynasty philosopher Zhu Xi when he exclaimed: "Today the profession of medicine is the noblest profession in the world . . . and the writing of eight-legged essays the basest."[3]

These basic ideas have led to a political consensus that has held through all China's administrations from the 1920s into the present. The original goal of resolving the situation by prohibiting Chinese medicine and starting from scratch with Western medicine was, however, never politically feasible. Nevertheless, the compromise position of a gradual suppression of Chinese medicine seemed practicable. The following chapters will note some of the more remarkable milestones of this development.

14

THE PERSUASIVENESS
OF WESTERN MEDICINE

Already by the eighteenth century, several stimuli had occurred that might have encouraged the Chinese to engage with European medicine. The French priest Father Parennin had prepared detailed anatomical plates for the Emperor Kangxi in 1722; the emperor immediately rejected them as unsuitable, so the original illustrations were sent back to France and may now be consulted in a Paris library. At the beginning of the nineteenth century, surgeons of the Dutch East India Company sought out contact with indigenous healers while they were stationed at Macao. At this time they were not burdened with a feeling of superiority: that came only after the 1830s.

The first revolution in European medicine came with the development of modern anesthetic methods, facilitating new surgical techniques. Shortly thereafter, knowledge of the chemical basis for active pharmacological principles set in motion the new pharmacology with its mass production of reliably effective drugs. Finally, the discovery of the causes of disease allowed for the possibility of therapies that could attack them directly inside the body and suggested external preventive measures before they reached the body.

At around the same time, Rudolf Virchow (1821–1902) published his book on "cellular pathology," thereby initiating research leading to the long-awaited synthesis between morphological findings and their chemical and physical significance for health and disease.

All of these changes occurred within half a century. The conceptual difference between modern European medicine near the end of the nineteenth century and its forerunner of the 1830s was of the same order of magnitude as the difference between the ubiquitous use of smart phones, tablet computers, and the Internet today and the use of slate tablets, soapstone pencils, and sponge erasers in schools as recently as the 1950s.

It is hard to imagine the level of enthusiasm for science that gripped the entire population at that time, since nowadays there are increasing questions about the legitimacy of modern medicine's exclusive attention to a physico-chemical worldview that focuses only on the material structures of the human organism. One must make an effort to put oneself in that environment in order to understand the increasing self-confidence with which doctors of Western medicine ventured out into the world, including to China, where they looked down condescendingly on the prescientific therapies of non-Western peoples. From the other side, many Chinese observers were gripped with the same enthusiasm.

Starting from the 1830s, British and American missionary societies promoted extra medical education for their missionaries, as a way of protecting their health and promoting their survival in the frequently insalubrious environments, beyond the reach of Western civilization, in which they were sent to work. In China it soon became clear that missionaries' medical knowledge gained more attention and created greater demand from the local population than evangelizing for the Christian gospel alone. Christianity appeared largely incomprehensible, whereas when Chinese encountered missionary medicine, it seemed much less strange. Minor surgical interventions were the most persuasive, as the relationship between intervention and effect was obvious to even lay observers.

A few of the missionaries acceded to the wishes of their Chinese assistants and instructed them in Western medicine, or sent them to Japan or the United States to get a regular education in medicine. On their return, the newly minted doctors compared the status of medicine in these foreign countries with the wretched conditions offered by the missionary hospitals in China, a comparison that ignited a storm of outrage. This motivated the Rockefeller Foundation to increase its financing of hospitals in China so that they could more closely emulate the model represented by the Johns Hopkins Hospital in Baltimore. The process culminated in the 1920s, when we can conclusively say that modern Western medicine had its beginning in China. The Peking Union Medical College, established by the Rockefeller Foundation in Beijing in 1921, has survived all the tribulations of the last hundred years and succeeded in maintaining the highest standards of medicine.

The rapid assimilation of Western individualized medicine was not only due to its therapeutic successes. Many of its concepts and therapeutic approaches were already familiar to at least the better-educated Chinese. The circulation of the blood, concepts of the body's own resistance to disease and of pathological influences that attacked from the outside to imperil an otherwise healthy organism, the Doctrine of the Mean—these and other aspects of Western medicine had their approximate equivalents in Chinese medical history and theory, even if not all of them were central to it. The aspects of Western medicine that required a more radical change of orientation were the emphasis on morphology and anatomy, the analytical sciences, and not least, the renunciation of respect for the models of the past. It required a conviction that only new research, which would approach the old traditions with skepticism, could provide increasingly effective knowledge about health and disease.

Additionally, before the encounter with Western civilization, there was absolutely no concept of a politics of "public health." In Europe in the late eighteenth century, new political structures arose, confronted with challenges that were unknown in China. In the process of putting the old feudal structures behind them, the countries of Europe now, for the first time, regarded themselves to a greater or lesser degree as national communities. The new nation-states competed in two ways. First, they competed with the productive forces of their manufactories, leading to rapid development of modern industries. The cornerstone of the productivity of these industries was a healthy, productive population, regardless of class, income, or education. All members needed to be strong and healthy; those "below" even more so than those "above" when working days of up to fourteen hours were commonplace.

The second pillar of successful competition among the new nation-states was the military. The wars associated with the French Revolution had convinced military strategists of the value of soldiers with a patriotic attitude. This led to a devaluation of the armies of mercenaries of the past. The new argument was that the more strong and healthy young men a state had at its disposal, the more readily it would be able to defend itself from external attacks, or the better it could successfully carry out such attacks on neighboring countries. Both politics and medicine reacted promptly with the concept of "public health" to these new realizations.

The idea of public health rested on an understanding that even though individuals can promote their own health in specific ways, this personal responsibility is frequently compromised by environmental, living, and working conditions. Once the mighty and the rich had recognized the detrimental impact of the limited ability

of individual citizens—in particular those of the lower classes—
to care for their health, on a country's productive and military
strength, they very soon listened to what advice medicine could
give. For the first time in two thousand years doctors were admon-
ished to go beyond appealing to individuals to live in healthy ways.
From now on they enjoyed a mandate also to admonish governments, industries, etc. to arrange each person's environment in
such a way that it would no longer be detrimental to their health.
Public health became a task to be fulfilled by society. This was the
starting point of European health policies. Without knowledge of
these historical facts, one will not understand why European countries were eventually eager and able to set up so-called "solidaristic
health insurance plans." Health in itself was not the primary goal,
but a means to an end. The goal was to create a particularly strong,
because healthy, social community: the state.

China had never before encountered this political compulsion
to treat the health of its inhabitants as a means to achieve a strong
state, which in turn would depend on the health of every individual. The idea of individual responsibility laid out in the basic theory
of traditional Chinese medicine—"My fate lies in my own hands,
not in Heaven"—is still considered valid; it has been expanded in
various ways only through the twentieth-century efforts to modern-
ize China.

The first time that public health, combined with modern science and epidemiology—another specialty previously unknown in
China—showed itself to be convincingly effective was in the battle
against the so-called "Manchurian plague" outbreak in 1910–1911. As
whole stretches of the landscape were depopulated and all traditional
methods of prevention and therapy proved useless, including, most
notably, attempts to exorcise the relevant disease demons, the Chinese authorities transferred responsibility for managing the epidemic to a British-educated Chinese microbiologist by the name

of Wu Lien-teh. Because of his Chinese ethnicity, Wu had been unable to get an official position in the government health administration of his homeland, the British colony of Malaya. Wu was schooled in the science of the day and consistently applied this knowledge to justify his efforts in epidemic disease control, eventually bringing the plague outbreak to an end.[1]

There could be no clearer indication of how the future health administration of China was to be organized. When in 1914, a delegation of Chinese-medical doctors came to appeal to the government to protect Chinese medicine from extinction, the education minister responsible for such issues, Wang Daxie, gave this unvarnished response: "I have decided in future to abolish Chinese medicine and also not to use Chinese drugs." When the delegation took their concerns on to the interior minister, they were greeted with an equally brusque dismissal.

15

THE OPINIONS OF INTELLECTUALS
AND POLITICIANS

Chen Duxiu (1879–1942) was one of the founders of the Chinese
Communist Party in 1921 and served as its first General Secretary.
He came from a wealthy family, and in the last years of imperial
rule he passed the first level of civil service examinations, coming
in first place. In spite of this he became a reformer with initially
social-democratic leanings but eventually, under the influence of
Marxist ideology, a revolutionary. He knew the West well and may
have studied for a while in France. His affection for France came to
an end at the termination of the First World War, however, when
France prevented the return of China's former German concessions to Chinese control, agreeing instead to have them transferred
to Japan. Chen Duxiu repeatedly expressed his unconditional trust
in Western science as the necessary means to facilitate China's recovery, as for example in his famous 1919 "Call to Youth," published
in the journal *New Youth* that he had founded in 1915:

> Our scholars know nothing of science; that is why they turn to the yin-
> yang signs and belief in the Five Phases in order to confuse the
> world and delude the people. . . . Our doctors know nothing of sci-
> ence; they know nothing of human anatomy and also have no idea

how to analyze drugs. They have not even heard of bacterial toxins and infections. . . . The pinnacle of their superstition is the theory of *qi*, which in fact belongs to the antics of street performers and Daoist priests. We can never comprehend this *qi*, even if we search for it throughout the whole universe. All these imaginary ideas and irrational beliefs can be thoroughly rectified with science. If we are to reach the truth with science, we must first verify all the facts. . . . There are no limits to truth in the universe, and in the realm of science there are vast fertile regions awaiting explorers to open them up. Youth, to work!

A long list of more or less radical reformers and revolutionaries from the ranks of intellectuals and also politicians could be enumerated here as agreeing with Chen Duxiu's opinions. Many of those who committed their dislike of Chinese medicine to paper, whether in literary or documentary form, were motivated by their own sorry experiences with it. Lu Xun (1881–1936), one of the most significant and influential Chinese authors of the twentieth century, dealt with some of his experiences in his short story "Medicine" (*Yao* 藥).

In this story, the son of a couple who run a teahouse is suffering from tuberculosis. When a young man from the same town is arrested by the authorities as a revolutionary on the basis of accusations by one of his relatives, the father of the sick child, following a tip, spends a great deal of money to buy a steamed bun dipped in the blood of the executed man from the executioner. He gives it to his son, believing it to be a guaranteed panacea. The son dies anyway. The story, which is rich in more or less hidden symbolism, was influenced by Lu Xun's experiences as a young man when he was required to fetch apparently ineffective traditional therapies from a distant pharmacy and even sent to gather herbs from allegedly especially suitable places to treat his father, who was sick for many years. The enormous cost of these treatments reduced the family to financial ruin, which eventually also contributed to Lu Xun having to give up his studies of Western medicine in Japan. As a result of his father's protracted martyrdom and the treatments proposed by his traditional-style doctors, Lu Xun was rendered incapable of any sympathy for Chinese medicine or its supporters. "Medicine" was one of his first published works of fiction, appearing in 1919 in *New Youth*. In his next short story, "Morning," he expressed himself even more clearly with the character of an incompetent doctor who, again, was responsible for the death of a child.

A little later, in 1922, director Zhang Shichuan released China's first slapstick film, *Laborer's Love* (*Lao gong zhi ai qing* 老工之愛 情). For a slapstick comedy film to succeed, it has to have a character universally regarded as ridiculous at the core of the story. Zhang Shichuan chose a doctor of Chinese medicine for this role. The doctor has so few patients he is unable to pay the rent for his roadside stall, so when a fruit seller asks for the hand of his daughter in marriage, he refuses, saying that he needs a son-in-law who can help him financially. The young man finally comes up with a plan: he rebuilds the stairs that lead to the bar above his simple lodgings so that he can temporarily manipulate them, causing the patrons to fall and suffer all kinds of injuries, which are then treated in various absurd ways by the father of his intended bride. This brings extra income to the doctor, who duly changes his mind and accepts the fruit seller as his son-in-law.

Ba Jin (1904–2005) was an author with anarchist political leanings who, like Lu Xun, used memories and impressions from his own upbringing to express his disdain for Chinese medicine. In spite of the fact that his writings were banned during the Cultural Revolution of the 1960s and 1970s, Ba Jin counts as one of the most widely read authors of the twentieth century in China. Because of this, the influence of his evaluation of both the past and the present on countless Chinese readers can hardly be overstated.

In his 1931 novel *Family* (*Jia* 家), Ba Jin addressed the contemporary conflict between two opposing forces: those who were prepared to hold fast to ancient Confucian social norms and structures even if this meant literally treading over dead bodies, and the younger generation eager to liberate themselves from the restrictions of convention. In his narrative, the author painted a complex portrait of traditional forms of healing that he held to be nonsensical and ultimately useless, describing a phalanx of incompetent representatives of classical medicine alongside folk healers and exorcists of demons, all of whom were supposed to help treat the ailments of the obstinate family patriarch.

Lao She (1899–1966) was the son of a Manchurian soldier who had been killed during the street fighting that accompanied the Boxer Rebellion of 1900. Despite his mother's poverty, Lao She was able to graduate with a teaching degree thanks to a college that waived tuition fees. Thereafter, he went to live in Europe and the United States, but returned to his homeland after the founding of the People's Republic of China in response to an invitation from Zhou Enlai. During the Cultural Revolution he was accused of being a reactionary and badly abused, escaping from his tormentors only by committing suicide. In his writings he described, often satirically, the conditions of the past in Beijing. This is the case in his 1933 story "Hugging a Grandson" (*Bao sun* 抱孫),[1] about the catastrophic ending of a pregnancy. A young couple decline the offer of a modern delivery in a hospital and instead entrust themselves to the superstitious procedures of the older generations. The author's message is unmistakeable: the old values are a fatal hindrance to the blessings of modern science and the medicine derived from it.

Ye Shaojun (1894–1988), as a final example, began his literary career as a writer of short stories in the classical style, then decided to contribute to the modernization of education for young people. He worked as a journalist for a long time, striving for a written style that was close to the spoken language and would be universally comprehensible. His descriptions of people's living conditions aimed to be as true to life as possible. In his story "A Posthumous Son" (*Yi fu zi* 遺腹子), he relates how a child's death is hastened by the use of Chinese medicine. His conclusion was that this medicine is more than useless: it is dangerous.

All these and many more condemnations of Chinese medicine threatened to drown out the efforts already under way by conservative doctors and their supporters to secure renewed support for traditional healing arts. The fact that Western medicine had never been able to offer cures for all diseases and often gave inferior results when compared with some methods practiced by many Chinese doctors was enough to ensure a continued strong demand for traditional healers. In politics, it was necessary to solve the dilemma of being committed to the modernization of China, yet not completely overlooking the needs and preferences of the people.

Many people, including medically trained authors, published suggestions for combining Western and Chinese medicine in some way. Proposals for reformulating Chinese medicine according to modern scientific criteria found approval from some people and vehement opposition from others who condemned Western medicine as an imperialist imposition and desired instead to see the essence of Chinese culture preserved in its traditional medicine. In the end, voices like those of Tan Zhuang gained the upper hand, for political reasons. He identified traditional Chinese medicine with the values of the old society, calling it "the medicine of the Confucian literati," and declared that "This so-called rich national essence is just the collected garbage of several thousand years."[2]

Chinese medicine remained disadvantaged in many respects until the mid-1950s. Doctors of Chinese medicine were urged to align their practices with those of modern medicine, which was a hopeless and unsuccessful undertaking. Finally, in 1954, Mao Zedong called for a change of approach. He handed over responsibility for the modernization of Chinese medicine to doctors trained in Western medicine. They were to study the clinical experiences of their Chinese medical colleagues, make sure they met the requirements of modern medicine, and finally combine Chinese and Western medicine into a single scientifically legitimate practice, which would simultaneously represent a new kind of world medicine. There was no doubt who was to be in charge of this combination process, as Mao stressed that "It is wrong for some to overemphasize the importance of Chinese medicine!"[3]

At the same time, the officials responsible for medical policy realized that the time had come to manage Chinese medicine's foreign relations. Already in the early 1950s, the Soviet Union and other nations of the Communist bloc had expressed interest in Chinese medicine. Other countries were also interested: two famous older doctors had received invitations to go to France to teach Chinese medicine there. The Chinese side had a large vested interest in being able to offer to the world a modernized Chinese medicine divested of all the fallacies and unscientific elements that had accompanied it in the past, and to provide this medicine with a designation that would evoke the impression of its continuity over thousands of years as a specifically Chinese culture of healing.

In 1955, these considerations led to the introduction of the English-language appellation "Traditional Chinese Medicine," usually abbreviated to TCM. This term was created solely for use in foreign-language publications; in Chinese the term *zhongyi*, literally "Chinese medicine," became the norm, displacing such previously equally common designations as "old-style medicine" and "national medicine." However, it would be another twenty years before the opening of China during the period of reform under Deng Xiaoping, and with it the worldwide spread of TCM as a kind of trademark, leading to the misconception that it was the equivalent of the premodern traditional practices, which plagues devotees of TCM to this day.

Just a few years after this Mao Zedong wrote a letter, one sentence of which led to a second, lasting misconception: "Chinese medicine and pharmacology constitute a great treasure-house." This sentence was cited for many years as a general expression of the great value Mao placed on traditional Chinese medicine. In fact, however, in its original context it was meant to express a much more limited, if not directly contradictory opinion. The sentence was included in a letter Mao wrote on October 11, 1958, to Yang Shangkun, who was Chairman of the General Office of the Central Committee of the Chinese Communist Party at the time. Mao was demanding the implementation of a program to send physicians of Western medicine to study traditional medicine. Each province, independent city, and autonomous region was required to enroll 70 to 80 doctors, so that after two or three years there would be about 2,000 doctors available who had augmented their Western-style medical education with traditional medicine and were competent in both: "Among these, there will probably emerge a few brilliant theoretical experts. . . . This is a major event and must not be taken lightly. Chinese medicine and pharmacy constitute a great treasure-house, and should be diligently explored and improved upon."[4]

In other words, in the history of Chinese medicine and pharmacy one could find many valuable elements that were to be assimilated into Western medicine and adapted so as to meet modern scientific standards. The rest of traditional medicine, and above all the traditional practitioners, were completely omitted from this evaluation.

16

THE SELECTION

Political attitudes toward the historical heritage of healing arts in the People's Republic of China (PRC) have been marked by various regulatory measures, heated debates, and the founding of dedicated institutions. Even though, when viewed from afar, the country seems obedient to an authoritarian regime, it is nonetheless clear that there has been a constant and significant current of resistance against the incessant forces of medical Westernization—a current that persists to this day. Despite all of the efforts and various slogans promoting the unification of Chinese with Western medicine, the stances of the participants have not softened. Standing at one side are the uncompromising modernizers, who have still not forgotten the trauma of China's humiliation at the hands of the superior science and technology of the West.

A recent attempt from this side to win the argument and invalidate the opposition came in the form of a demand to "Bid Farewell to Chinese Medicine" by Zhang Gongyao 張功耀, published on September 8, 2006. Zhang Gongyao is a professor of philosophy at Zhongnan University in Wuhan, and published his opinion piece in the journal *Medicine and Philosophy* "in the name of cultural progress, in the name of science, in the name of biodiversity, and in the name of humanity." The arguments provoked by his article are not materially different from those that took place in the first half of the twentieth century.

Intellectuals like Zhang Gongyao were voicing their opposition to conservative forces in society that remain powerful enough that Zhang felt the heat of their ire in the spirited debate that followed the publication of his article. The opposition's arguments were also not fundamentally different from those of a century ago, when the controversy began.

The decisive point here is that the development of Chinese medicine in the PRC has not been directed by physicians or other health care professionals relying on their own personal observations of patients or on scientific studies to advance medical knowledge. As described by the German sinologist, physician, and also practitioner of traditional Chinese medicine Barbara Volkmar, TCM is an "artificially systematic product"—a deliberately constructed system of concepts and practices that did not arrive at their present state through a process of historical development, but rather through the political calculations of responsible officials of the PRC.[1] This is particularly evident in the reorganization of acupuncture. The question of whether there exist such things as the bodily conduits to transport blood and vapors (*qi*) around the body, described over two thousand years ago, and the questions about where acupuncture points should be located were ultimately decided by political negotiation.

An influential contributor to the creation of a "New Acupuncture" was a modern physician by the name of Zhu Lian (1909–1978). Working in the context of the civil war/war of liberation of the 1940s, she viewed acupuncture as an extension of the battlefield into each individual organism. The terminology of her new acupuncture was accordingly borrowed from the military vocabulary of wartime. She saw no evidence for the existence of "conduits" of *qi*. In the place of the traditional practice of graphically representing these conduits by drawing lines between acupuncture points, she drew areas of the body, each defined by boundary lines that connected acupuncture points sharing similar effects, and given names that resembled the terminology for the communist base areas located away from enemy territory. The reworkings of traditional acupuncture proposed by Zhu Lian were so radical that it is hardly surprising that they failed to catch on. The end result was a negotiated compromise first seen in the education of acupuncturists in China and since extended worldwide.

The "excavation and recovery" of the gems in the "treasure trove of Chinese medicine" took place on different levels. Of the various conceptual systems of the Chinese past, the only explanatory model to be considered was the model of systematic correspondence. This had the benefit of being secular and could be reduced to a small number of core concepts, which although appearing exotic from the point of view of modern science, nonetheless did not directly offend modern sensibilities. The next step was to select from among the miscellaneous population of traditional healers, with their highly diverse educational backgrounds and varying levels of competency, only those who could be trusted to bring the practice of traditional medicine to a more advanced level. To this end, examinations were held to qualify traditional healers in 1953. The results were sobering. Only a tiny proportion met the requirements. And finally, there was the isue of how to organize the complex field of historical pharmacy. The *materia medica* texts of imperial China described the actions and effects of more than 2,000 natural and man-made substances. Their effectiveness was supposedly shown by their inclusion in innumerable recipe books. It was clear that there was much useful experiential knowledge in these sources to be "excavated and recovered," as Mao had put it, but much of it could not be assimilated into the new conceptual framework.

Examples of medical formulas that fell victim to the reorganization are given below. They are taken from pharmaceutical texts dating from the eighth to the sixteenth century, having survived on account of their reputations as tried-and-true remedies:

- For food stuck in the gullet: take shade-dried feces of macaque monkeys, roast it to ashes, and mix together with good wine. Administer this liquid and it will be effective in ten attempts or less.
- For a tendency to suffer nightmares and the absence of dreams: take the ashes of an incinerated corpse and place them in a headrest or in a shoe. This will stop it.
- Recipe for female sterilization: Take a one-foot-square piece of old paper made from silkworm eggs, burn it, and rub the ashes into powder. If a woman consumes these ashes dissolved in wine, she will be unable to bear children for the rest of her life.
- For sores on the eyebrows: take the roasted feces from a black donkey, grind them into powder, mix with oil, and apply to the sores. This will be immediately effective.
- Growths and warts: catch at least ten spiders from the flowering heads of rice plants and put them on peach tree twigs. Wait until they have spun threads that hang down from the twigs and collect the threads from the east side only. Spin the filaments together to make a thicker thread and use this to bind around the base of the growths or warts. Change the threads every few days, until the growths or warts fall off of their own accord.
- For chronic sadness and crying brought on by hearing someone else crying or sadness brought on by one's own crying that does not resolve itself spontaneously: scrape the dirt from between the teeth of a comb and ingest it with water.
- For spontaneous muscle bleeding: roast the hair from a fetus to ashes and apply to the wound. It will stop the bleeding.

- Children crying during the night: burn pig feces to ashes. Soak them in water, and filter this to obtain a juice that is then used to wash the child. At the same time, have the child ingest a small amount.
- For severe burns: take the head of a dead rat and cook it in pork fat that was collected during the twelfth month until the head has completely dissolved. To be applied externally.
- For a growth on the lip: take one *sheng* of pig excrement, mix it with water, and strain it through a piece of cloth. Drink the filtrate warm.
- For bedwetting: take the tips from twenty-seven hemp-straw shoes, roast them to ashes, and drink the ash mixed with spring water on the first day of the new year in the early morning.
- For discharges: burn felt to ashes and consume two *qian* mixed with wine. For white discharges, use white felt; for red discharges, use red felt.
- Nosebleeds: menstrual bleeding that directs itself upward.
- For internal blood stasis after childbirth: to treat obstructed blood in a woman who has given birth, collect black soot from the underside of a cooking pan and administer two *qian* of it mixed with wine.

This is only a small sampling: the list could be multiplied many times. I have given examples of recipes exhibiting the doctrine of magical correspondence, taken from the great recipe compendia of "regular" Chinese medicine. They persisted for many centuries and can mostly be found in texts that are regularly reprinted even today. Since the inscription in 2012 of the *Ben cao gang mu* on "the Memory of the World International Register" by UNESCO, some of them are now ennobled with this "world memory" designation.

Even within the core of the medicine of systematic correspondence, there are numerous theoretical explanations and therapeutic interventions for which no modern justification can be offered. Two examples from traditional ophthalmology will suffice to illustrate this fact. The first comes from a classical ophthalmological text ascribed to the Tang-dynasty doctor Sun Simiao but actually first compiled in the fifteenth and sixteenth centuries. This text, the *Yin hai jing wei*, describes how to treat an eye complaint known in Chinese medicine as *tou zhen*. In modern medical dictionaries, this complaint, which literally translates as "invisible needle," is glossed as *hordeolum* or, in common parlance, a stye.

Question: "When someone is suffering from a stye on the lower eyelid—which people refer to as an 'invisible needle'—what is happening?" Answer: "This is a case of heat poison in the yang-brightness conduit of the stomach. It is caused either by indulging in foods of an excessively hot nature, or simply eating and drinking to excess. This causes rising [of heat poison] along the lung conduit until it fills the eyes. As a consequence a toxic lesion often develops in the lower eyelid or in the corner of the eye. This is called 'an invisible needle.' To treat such cases, one should pull the lower lid down, puncture the lesion and allow the stagnant blood to escape. 'Cooling powder' should be applied directly to the site of the lesion, and then instruct [the patient] to take 'Redness-reducing powder,' followed by 'powder to unblock the essence' and 'liquid to drain the spleen.'"[2]

The second example is concerned with observations, understandings, and treatments of "epidemic red eye." Ophthalmologists today identify this disease as epidemic conjunctivitis and corneal inflammation on the basis of the same features described here: its high infectiousness, immunity to repeat infections, predictable course, and observable symptoms.

"Epidemic red eye" refers to the ability of poisonous *qi* flowing between heaven and earth to spread among the people. If one person's eyes are affected, that person will spread it to the entire family; all, regardless of age, will be affected at once. This is called "epidemic red eye." The swelling, pain, sandy roughness, and difficulty opening [the eyes] will be cured after about five days, since it is caused by the *qi* of one five-day period; thereafter the illness comes to an end.

Treatment: this condition must certainly not be needled or rinsed; merely boil *huang lian* [*Rhizoma coptidis*] in boy's urine, let it stand overnight, and rinse [the eyes] with the warm liquid five times a day in order to release the toxic influences. Then finely grind together *hu lian* [*Rhizoma picrorhizae*] and *xuan lian* [*Rhizoma coptidis* from Xuan prefecture] with *ku fan* [alum: potassium aluminum sulfate] and *xionghuang* [realgar: arsenic sulfide], mix the powder with fresh ginger juice, and put drops of this mixture into the corners of both eyes. When it touches there will be copious tears and the pain will stop immediately.[3]

To avoid misunderstanding, let me explain that these examples are not meant to represent the entirety of historical Chinese medicine; rather, they are presented here as some of the most striking illustrations of the fact that this medicine, just like the healing arts in the history of Europe, contained more than just rational observations and useful therapeutic tips. In fact, there were many therapies, medicinal recipes, and concepts of illness that would no longer be appropriate for clinical use; nowadays they appear absurd and even harmful.

The fact that we could find similar numbers of comparable examples in European pharmacy and recipe books from the past few centuries is, however, irrelevant, since the course of European medical and pharmaceutical history is well known and nobody denies it. Western medicine prides itself on subjecting its therapies to continual investigation, and when warranted, exchanging them for new and better treatments. This is not the case with the mythological "traditional

Chinese medicine." The myth is based on the idea of a system of medicine that is still useful in spite of being thousands of years old, unique, and the result of an unbroken chain of transmission from antiquity to the present. This myth is inaccurate, as can be clearly deduced from Mao's directive to "excavate and recover" those elements of Chinese medicine that were rational and useful. Opinions about what constituted the rational and useful elements to be excavated and recovered clearly differed greatly.

The conclusions drawn by those responsible for managing this heterogenous heritage followed a rationale that had long proved its effectiveness. Simply to forbid the practice of Chinese medicine with a stroke of a legislative pen was neither necessary from a professional standpoint nor economically justified, and in any case would have been politically unenforceable. So the political line adopted the objective of retaining those aspects of Chinese medicine that were considered useful and, as far as possible, legitimating them on the basis of modern scientific studies. The effects of this can be clearly seen in the education of the next generations of Chinese doctors of TCM.

Young people who aspire to become doctors are assigned to study modern Western medicine or TCM based on their university entrance examination results. The best students are admitted to modern medical schools; those who perform less well are assigned to colleges of Chinese medicine. Students of TCM are first trained in the basics of modern anatomy, pathology, and physiology, and are then required to study selected elements of Chinese medical theory. This orientation away from the context of modern culture and into the ancient concepts and thought processes of Chinese medicine requires serious effort and engagement. In this age of tablets and smart phones, college teachers from both mainland China and Taiwan report that motivating high school graduates to undertake this intellectual journey is becoming more and more difficult. They are scarcely better able to grasp the concept of *qi* than their contemporaries in the Western world. The supposed advantage of "being Chinese" and therefore benefiting from a culturally mediated access to the world of thought of premodern China is shrinking from year to year. For the youth of today, this cultural past is already very distant and foreign.

17

THE SURPRISE

In 1971, American journalist James Reston happened to be in southern China when he learned of U.S. Secretary of State Henry Kissinger's visit to China. Sensing that this might be an important movement in U.S.-Chinese relations, he applied for permission to travel to Beijing. The Chinese authorities approved his request but put him on a slow train so that he arrived three days too late to cover Kissinger's visit, which was in preparation for the state visit of President Richard Nixon the next year. In Beijing, Reston fell ill with appendicitis. He consented, after the successful operation, to the suggestion by his Chinese doctors to treat his postoperative pains with acupuncture, a therapy he had previously never heard of. He recorded his experiences, and *The New York Times* published his report on the front page on July 26, 1971. Shortly thereafter, the CIA sent at least one agent to investigate and report on the military potential of this new method of "anesthesia"—which as we know now provides at best only partial analgesia—as it seemed to require no complicated operating room setup, and hence was a promising candidate for medical field operations in locations of military activity where electricity might be lacking.

Needle therapy had been familiar to only a very small circle of doctors and healers in Europe and the United States up to that point; now this changed overnight. Hordes of doctors, politicians, alternative healers, and laypeople traveled to China in increasing numbers to inform themselves about traditional healing methods. For their part, the Chinese were completely astonished by the flood of Western interest. As a deputy minister for research recalled, in conversation with the author: "We simply could not understand how it was that Westerners, who had already experienced the Renaissance and the Enlightenment and who were committed to scientific knowledge, suddenly became enthusiastic about these old things!"

The visitors from the West were graciously received and introduced to TCM—not, of course, to the historical multiplicity of Chinese healing arts, but rather to the minor "artificial systematic product" of "Traditional Chinese Medicine." For Western students, that was already exotic enough. The basic concepts of systematic correspondence in the explanatory framework of yin and yang and the Five Phases were both foreign and yet at the same time easy to comprehend. The really challenging aspects of these theories were no longer to be found in TCM, at least not by beginners; the logical foundations had already been thoroughly aligned with Western patterns of thought. The teachings that these early visitors to China took back home with them were vague enough to be open to all kinds of individual interpretations. Above all, they were well suited to representing whatever opposing views the student had been seeking as correctives to the perceived shortcomings of their own biomedicine.

On the Chinese side, however, there was ambivalence. Nobody had been able to anticipate the fact that the Westerners would value TCM primarily as an alternative to Western medicine, a situation we shall explore in more detail below. As the misunderstanding became ever more evident, and the Chinese were forced to accept that TCM in the West had taken on a political meaning that was the direct opposite of the meaning intended by the Chinese leadership, they started to take steps to ameliorate the situation. Acupuncture societies in the West were offered cooperative agreements with Chinese colleges and internships in Chinese hospitals in return for their acceptance of Chinese interpretations of acupuncture and therapeutics. In 2007 the Chinese government invited ministers of science and health from around the world to come to China to work on and then adopt the "Beijing Declaration on Traditional Chinese Medicine." This was a pre-prepared document that was presented to the delegates to be discussed and then finally endorsed.

The key messages to be driven home to the foreign ministers were: "TCM is a form of medicine fully grounded in modern biological science" and "The future of TCM lies in molecular biology." This was a clear statement that the conventional and historical explanatory systems of Chinese medicine were going to be completely replaced at some unstated future date. While Chinese cultural propaganda continues to pay generous lip service to the historical value and ancient concepts of traditional Chinese medicine, the actual political developments have continued along a single trajectory: the modernization of TCM to the point of complete assimilation with Western medicine. This goes hand in hand with continued efforts to get legal approval for export to Europe of patent remedies created from traditional formulas. While all of this goes on in the name of TCM, it has precious little in common with the Chinese medicine of the past.

18

THE CREATIVE RECEPTION OF
CHINESE MEDICINE IN THE WEST

Anyone wishing to find out about traditional Chinese medicine these days is likely to rely on information gleaned from the Internet by entering relevant search terms into a search engine such as Google. Doing this brings up entries such as these:

Asian medicine, particularly the traditional healing arts of China, are among humanity's oldest forms of medicine. Already several thousand years ago, wise Chinese recognized that particular forms of energy flow to all parts of the body. The pathways of this energy, which lie below the skin, are known as meridians. If this vital flow of energy is interrupted at one or more locations, health problems are the result. In this, Chinese medicine recognizes the only interpretation of disease for which it alone can provide effective treatment.

Traditional Chinese Medicine.
    Traditional Chinese Medicine, abbreviated as TCM, draws from a history of more than 3,000 years. According to legend, it was founded by the two Emperors Shen Nong and Huang Di. The former is reputed to have taught the people how to use healing herbs, while the latter introduced needle treatment to medical practice. The most important

principles of Chinese medicine are the theories of yin and yang and the Five Phases or Elements, along with the theory of *qi*, the universal vital force and energy.

Welcome to a new and fascinating world. Chinese treatment methods—which are simultaneously new and over 2,000 years old—have only recently attracted public interest in Switzerland. Chinese medicine is based on the philosophy of Daoism, and fascinates us with its gentle and natural diagnosis and treatment methods that have been recognized for several hundred years.

Chinese medicine: what is it, actually?
    Chinese medicine (CM) is an autonomous medical system that is about 6,000 years old and that emerged out of the background of Daoist teachings. In the course of its long history, it had periods of varying medical quality. People repeatedly strove to render the ancient principles more tangible, and to organize CM systematically, so that it could remain compatible with new developments. In the 1950s, the Chinese government decided to lend its strong support to CM even though it was almost defunct at the time, and began to found academies for CM. In this period of the "revitalization" of CM, an abridged version was compiled that included material from classical texts.

The prize entry so far can be found at a website for managers that provides information leaving no further room for dispute:

The roots of traditional Chinese medicine can be traced back around 10,000 years. The written tradition is about 2,000 years old, and still today the "Yellow Emperor's Canon of Inner Phenomena" is used as a standard text. It contains the entirety of the knowledge of TCM.
    Increasing numbers of regular doctors are using a combination of Western and traditional Chinese medicine to meet the needs and

desires of their patients to be viewed as whole human beings and not just as a clinical picture composed of different symptoms.

What is behind TCM?

It is important to understand that TCM is a holistic medicine that views each person as a unitary combination of bodily spirit and soul. It is based on Daoist natural philosophy, on empirical observations of people, and on laboratory experiments.

All parts of the body, organs, and functional systems are connected with each other through the so-called meridians, or energy pathways. If this energy is able to flow unhindered through these pathways around the body, the person is in harmony with themselves and with the environment.

It is clear that the imagination of these authors knows no bounds. A few of those who offer instruction in theoretical and practical TCM seem to want to outbid each other in their estimations of the length of its history, as though the age of the practice were a significant marker of its quality. The appeal of Daoism exceeds that of Confucianism for Westerners who are inspired by alternative lifestyles. Therefore it is necessary to associate TCM with Daoism. Chinese practitioners who come to the West are not usually familiar with the correct catchwords to use in order to achieve the best response from this clientele. So it is highly unlikely that any doctor or health care practitioner in the West would come up with the idea of connecting the origins of TCM with demonic healing. In China, it is quite the opposite. Even today in China there is widespread agreement that demonic healing, TCM, and modern science all have their value. We should therefore not be surprised to find a Chinese who describes her practice as the "Berlin clinic of a health practitioner and China-certified head physician," blithely offering her personal opinion of the origins of TCM on her website, even though it flies in the face of both local knowledge and the historical facts:

> The earliest influences on TCM date from Chinese antiquity in about 2600 B.C.E. These included knowledge of how to read oracles, something that has become popular in the modern West with the popularity of the *Yijing* (I Ching), and demonic medicine, among others. In ancient China, beginning in about 1030 B.C.E., the main influences on traditional Chinese medicine were the two new philosophical approaches of Daoism and Confucianism. Both of these now constitute the foundations of TCM. The Zhou dynasty (1066–256 B.C.E.) saw important developments in medicine with precise descriptions of the human body and its diseases.

The educational system in the People's Republic of China, even at the elementary level, is not so poor that any observant pupil would not immediately know that Confucius's teachings could hardly have contributed to the development of TCM several centuries before the sage was even born, just as Daoism was not yet in existence to influence the medicine of the eleventh century B.C.E. One is left to wonder what the Chinese "head physician" intended to convey to her potential patients in Berlin with the text cited above. There are many similar examples to be found on the Internet; we need not explore them further. Even German doctors can be found publishing imaginative accounts such as the following, which informed readers of the *Deutsche Ärzteblatt* (German medical news) in 2004 that:

> Acupuncture is a harmonious equilibrium of forces. It is an ancient Chinese understanding that originating in the Dao, the mysterious origin of the universe, the vital force *qi* pervades, as "origin *qi*," the entire cosmos. This *qi* includes the two opposites yin and yang. All aspects

of the universe are composed of these two opposing elements or principles. For every yin there is an opposing yang. With the union of yin and yang it is possible to achieve complete harmony within a continuously changing whole.

Here is a further example, posted on the Internet by another German doctor of biomedicine:

Chinese medicine, which is one of the oldest human medical traditions, has been practiced successfully for thousands of years. It is based on an absolutely coherent theory of nature, even if this theory is foreign to Western understanding. Traditional Chinese Medicine operates on principles of analogy. That is, it correlates biological processes based on their mutual correspondences. In Chinese medicine the mode of reasoning is not through linear cause-effect relationships but rather in terms of multidimensional networks and circles of influence. In this way it benefits from a broader perspective and can draw on the subjective experiences of patients as well as on objectively ascertainable findings in making diagnoses.

What is questionable here is not so much the representation of this personal point of view as the treatment of the historical facts. Where, we may ask, did the author of these lines gather his information about the historical realities of Chinese medicine? Who told him that Chinese medical reasoning is "not through linear cause-effect relationships"? Where did he study Western medicine and learn that the subjective experiences of patients are neglected and not taken into account in making diagnoses? Perhaps he was thinking of patients such as a woman known to me who suffered from diarrhea for over a week and after a thorough investigation was informed by her biomedical physician, "Nothing is wrong with you!" She then took herself to a practitioner of TCM, who was able to resolve the issue using an entirely conventional Chinese-style interpretation and treatment. There are many similar cases that one could cite, but they do not add up to the blanket generalizations about Chinese and Western medicine offered here.

If the quotations given above constituted only isolated cases, there would be no reason to highlight them. But in fact, anyone with an Internet connection who enters the necessary search terms will find themselves confronted with an almost infinite number of comparable entries. Of course, there can be no objection when physicians, healers, and laypeople who are frustrated with the many shortcomings of Western medicine are motivated to look for ways to improve on them. A perusal of the tables of contents of the *German Journal of Acupuncture* from the past several years gives the decided impression that a majority of ailments, internal and otherwise, can and should be successfully treated with needle therapies. This may seem to be the case from the point of view of practitioners, but it does not justify the kind of grotesque historical falsification used to extoll TCM as the ideal alternative. As an example, in July 2011 the President of the Technical University of Munich awarded the title of Honorary Professor to a German physician who was celebrated in the press because he had "played a decisive role in shaping traditional Chinese medicine in Germany."[1] And this even though he had never read a single text in the original Chinese and knew nothing of the history of Chinese medicine! Those famous critics such as Lu Xun, Ba Jin, and the countless other Chinese who turned to this medicine over the course of the centuries in hopes of treatment and instead received malpractice would have wondered whether they had landed in an alternate universe if they had the opportunity to compare their experiences with the following characterization:

Our Western medicine places the material, the organic, at the center of analysis. From the viewpoint of traditional Chinese physicians, the individual is regarded—generally speaking—as an "embodiment of energetics." The human being is the reflection of the natural harmonies stretching between heaven and earth, between the poles of *yin* and *yang*. A Chinese doctor is interested in the "energetic phenomena," the active manifestations of life, the emotions, the vital bodily functions, because these will indicate the possible disharmonies of the "energetic structure" of the individual human being. Because traditional doctors take note of all the information that is available to them, thereby honoring the patient's whole person, there is consequently no place or reason for any distinction between psyche and soma, mind and body.

And it goes on. How we are to apply this "embodiment of energetics" to the training and appropriate treatment of, for example, a stye in the eye or a case of cervical cancer in a pregnant woman is never explained. We are justified in asking how it is possible, in this age of unprecedented access to information, to get away with such a complete disregard for the historical facts.

We can trace the beginnings of these myths and legends to two developments: in the first half of the twentieth century, a Frenchman by the name of Georges Soulié (1878–1955), who changed his name to George Soulié de Morant in order to give the appearance of belonging to the nobility, published his book *L'Acuponcture Chinoise*. It had enormous influence, first in France and then in the rest of the world. The second development came in the 1970s, when China unexpectedly opened its borders and presented its Traditional Chinese Medicine to an astonished world.

Soulié de Morant's book was an enormous achievement. Where he acquired the bits and pieces of his knowledge of Chinese medicine remains unclear—it was likely not from China, even though he lived there for several years.[2] Soulié de Morant had a good knowledge of Chinese but was less well informed about historical Chinese medicine. Two aspects of his writings have outlived him and spread throughout Western literature on Chinese medicine—they have, in fact, "decidedly influenced" traditional Chinese medicine in Europe and eventually the entire Western world, and played a part in distancing it from the Chinese original.

The first of these is his name for the internal conduits through which the ancient Chinese envisaged the flow of vapors (qi) and blood: he called them "meridians." This name suggested itself after he saw Chinese models of the body with the paths of the inner conduits painted on the outside, rather like the meridians painted on globes of the earth. The term "meridian" is completely unsuitable and misguided, but nonetheless it has become a standard translation.

Soulié de Morant's second, and far more problematic legacy, affecting first acupuncture and then TCM in general, is his definition of the concept of qi as "energy." There is no evidence of a concept of "energy"—either in the strictly physical sense or even in more colloquial senses—anywhere in Chinese medical theory. Many meanings have been associated with qi over the course of time, but to equate qi with "energy" is a European projection. It was nonetheless eagerly accepted in China, as it suggested that TCM was grounded in modern science. This interpretation of qi as energy was initially restricted to a relatively small circle of adherents, primarily in France, until the confluence of two developments in the 1970s: the global energy crisis and the simultaneous opening of China.

The opening of China after the state visit of U.S. President Nixon in 1972 was a surprise to Western observers. Behind the scenes, Kissinger had been making preparations for many months, but these had not been shared with the general public. When James Reston described his experiences in a front-page article in *The New York Times,* it did not take long for the U.S. government to send a team of doctors to China to report. They were soon followed by private parties. The people who were first on the scene inquired of their official guides and interpreters and were given the official versions of acupuncture and TCM. They took these official explanations and reported them back home and soon after also in Europe, where their testimony had enormous influence even though they knew no Chinese, had no knowledge of the history of medicine in China, and had had no long-term opportunities to witness the actual practice of Chinese medicine.

This characterization also applies to the authors of the first best-selling books about Chinese medicine, whose writings were highly instrumental in shaping the image of TCM in the West. First among these was Ted Kaptchuk. Kaptchuk, who is now a professor at Harvard Medical School researching the mechanisms of the placebo effect, wrote the first best-seller about TCM, *The Web That Has No Weaver*. In the introduction to this book, he wrote that causality is only of secondary importance in Chinese medicine, and that ideas of networked connections and simultaneity are much more important and constitute the essential characteristics of Chinese medicine. [3] Even though this description is not historically accurate, it met with a sympathetic reception in the West. It completely overlooked such fundamental writings as Chen Yan's twelfth-century monograph, *Formulas Organized According to the Three Types of Causes Underlying All Diseases*, and took no notice of the opinions of many other historical physicians on the meanings of disease causality, for example, those of Xu Dachun.

The book was published at a time and zeitgeist when growing numbers of especially younger people in the United States and Europe were engaged in the search for a cosmology that would account for all kinds of phenomena in a new and holistic way. All of a sudden, a message spread in the West that nothing that happens on the globe can be traced to a single final cause. All events and phenomena are interrelated. The movement of a butterfly's wings in the Amazon jungle may eventually lead to a storm in Norway. It was the beginning of a new era in Western mentality, and the characterization offered by Ted Kaptchuk put his construct of Chinese medicine exactly at the center of the resulting quest for holism, not only in world and local politics but also in our management of health and disease.

Kaptchuk rejected the one-to-one correspondence between *qi* and energy: he preferred to identify it as "a condition somewhere between energy and matter," whatever that might mean in concrete terms.[4] In fact, the influence of Soulié de Morant was already visible. TCM would be increasingly marketed as a healing art that placed the energetic causes of human disease at its center. The anxieties that had been unleashed by the energy crises of the 1970s had found their medical-theoretical cure. In the meantime there was also a ready audience in Germany for Chinese practitioners who claimed to employ ancient exorcistic talismans "to cleanse the body and the environment from poisons" and "to disperse the negative energy in foodstuffs and beverages."

An example of a German contribution to the creative reception of Chinese medicine in the West is furnished by the late Munich University professor of Chinese studies Manfred Porkert (1933–2015). His contribution came right at the beginning of Western interest in this previously unknown healing art and endured for a considerable period. Porkert had studied with some of the most celebrated scholars of Chinese culture in Paris, but he neglected to take the time to inform himself sufficiently about the history of Chinese medicine. His enthusiasm for his subject led him too quickly to assertions about the uniqueness of TCM that cannot be substantiated, or at best are only marginally supported by the historical facts.

In order to better express his conviction that Chinese medical terminology was at least as precise as the technical terminology of

Western medicine, Porkert translated classical Chinese medical terms with corresponding terms from Latin and ancient Greek. A few examples will suffice to illustrate the effects of this: for "acupuncture points," *xue* 穴 (literally "caves," "holes"), he used *foramina*; if these lay on the network vessels, he called them *foramina nexoria*. The long-term storage organs, *zang*, he translated as "function circle" and gave the Latin term *orbis*. The term *zang xiang*, the "externally observable signs of the condition of an internal long-term storage organ," was rendered in his highly sophisticated terminological system as "orbisiconography." The "visitor *qi*," *ke qi* 客氣, of pathology was likewise translated as *Ch'i deversans*. And so on. There were consequences to these choices.

The colloquial expressions of medical Chinese and the images they convey are important for understanding the relationship of ancient Chinese medicine to its political and institutional context. These disappeared in what was, for most readers, a highly abstract terminology. In this, Porkert contributed significantly to the estrangement of Chinese medicine in Western translation from its original cultural context. In addition, because of his lack of understanding of the metaphorical meanings of the original terminology, Porkert misidentified important concepts. For example, because he failed to appreciate that the yin-yang pair of *yingqi*, stationed troops *qi*, and *weiqi*, guard *qi*, referred to static and mobile protective *qi* in the human body, he glossed them as *Ch'i constructivum*, or "constructive energy," and *Ch'i defensivum*, or "defensive energy."[5]

Even more concerning was his rendering of *xie qi* 邪氣, literally "evil *qi*," as *Ch'i heteropathicum*. Instead of using the literal translation of *xie qi* as "evil *qi*" in English, many authors have based their translations on Porkert's, so that the term "heteropathic *qi*" has become commonplace in English publications on TCM. This has led to the loss of the entire context from the original Chinese term, the meaning of which depends on the contrast between *xie*, "evil, heterodox, false, misguided, depraved," and *zheng* 正, "righteous, orthodox, correct, upright." Porkert's antonyms of *Ch'i heteropathicum* and *Ch'i orthopathicum* give readers little indication of the degree to which Chinese physiology and pathology are deeply embedded in a wide-ranging set of dichotomous moral categories.

Porkert also contrasted the deductive reasoning that is supposedly dominant in Western medicine with what he characterized as the "inductive-synthetic" methodology of Chinese medical theorists. Even though there were a few objections to some of Porkert's blanket generalizations, such as "the scientific medicine of the West is based exclusively on the causal-analytical mode of cognition, whereas scientific Chinese medicine is based on an inductive-synthetic mode of cognition,"[6] the general enthusiasm for TCM worked to promote such black-and-white comparisons. The impressive multiplicity of Chinese theoretical approaches, many of them overlapping, has been excluded from many subsequent discussions. What has taken priority is the creation of equivalences between a generalized Chinese medicine and a particular characteristic.

Porkert's Latin terminology created an impenetrable barrier to communication with the homeland of TCM and acupuncture, so its use has been restricted to a fringe group of TCM practitioners who still adhere to Porkert's teachings, reading his *Sermons* and thereby promoting the creation of partisan sects within TCM.[7]

It is certainly understandable that a German physician and author would find the material emphasis of conventional medicine inadequate to meet the demands of his practice. After all, similar conclusions were reached by the anthroposophists in Germany more than a hundred years ago. One can also scarcely object when someone picks, from the history of Chinese medicine, any prescientific concepts, reformulates them according to modern knowledge into a new theory of physiology and pathology, and then labels this newly created mode of healing "energy medicine." What is not legitimate is to project these preferences onto the entirety of Chinese medicine and to claim it as a homogenous, superior culture of medicine when compared with the equally homogenous, but inadequate medicine of the West.

Not least, with respect to such claims, one has the right to ask: Why there is no evidence to suggest that the Chinese population enjoyed better health before the encounter with Western medical culture, or that they lived longer than their less privileged European contemporaries? And why was the Chinese population, which must have been so much more familiar with the traditional culture of China and therefore with the supposed advantages of this culturally embedded medicine, still so eager to take advantage of Western medicine with all of its deficiencies, in spite of the many dire warnings from the West?

TCM in the West has become, in many ways, a belief system deriving legitimacy from several different modes of exegesis, and entirely divorced from the reality of its historical past. When a Swiss citizen, writing on an Internet forum, expresses the opinion that some medical realities are not accessible to modern scientific methods, he is—like so many others—giving his personal interpretation of history and in doing so is rendering TCM unfalsifiable, in much the same way as is commonplace for religious belief systems:

> Academic evaluations of TCM from a purely rational perspective are bound to do it injustice. This system of medicine is based on a very different philosophy and on a completely different definition of reality that includes intuition, emotions, and instinct in addition to intellectual understanding. Just take the concept of freely flowing qi energy as the basis of good health: this is something that cannot be demonstrated with Western science.[8]

The adherents of the various interpretations bring their own worldviews and preferences, in each case based on their own experiences, accidental encounters, and the type of education they have had. The spectrum is wide. At one end are those who are strongly critical of the "cherry-picking" political approach of the People's Republic of China, who consider the disregard of so many historical concepts as a great loss and deem the attempt to merge Chinese medicine with modern medicine a pointless endeavor. At the other end of the spectrum are physicians who seek to connect modern neuroanatomical understandings of pain, organ failure, and mental illness with ancient Chinese concepts of *qi* circulation and organ function, in order that they may treat soldiers who are suffering from physical and mental trauma with their ear and scalp acupuncture on the basis of classical conduit theory.

Reliable criteria by which to judge the merits of the different factions are lacking. At the moment there is no prospect of a single institution large enough to bring the various currents of TCM practice together and create a synthesis worthy of the title "traditional Chinese medicine." Some schools are willing to enter into coalitions with each other, while others maintain a splendid isolation, certain of their unique possession of the true, "classical" or "canonical" Chinese medicine.

19

THE OBJECTIFICATION
OF THE DISCUSSION

Opportunity and Challenge

The situation we find ourselves in certainly has its positive aspects. Never before has there been an era of such unprecedented therapeutic freedom as exists today. And never have so many therapeutic approaches been able to compete for public favor. What is still lacking, however, is an objective means of differentiating which basic values should be endorsed in the emergent structure of any new health system. Such differentiation must start with recognition of the facts. For one, it requires the recognition and acceptance of the trust issues experienced by people who are unwilling to have their health problems treated only with modern biomedicine, with its novel diagnostic and therapeutic technologies and its modern pharmaceuticals. In this sector of the patient population, the repeated critiques and even polemics that appear in the print media against scientifically unproven statements and scientifically unverifiable therapeutic promises on behalf of Chinese medicine and other "alternative" healing practices seem to go unheeded. This brings up a fundamental question.

How can it be justified in the twenty-first century, in regard to our culturally and philosophically increasingly heterogenous population, to ask them to put aside their emotions in precisely that most sensitive area of human existence—the encounter with illness, disability, and the prospect of an early death—and instead to allow themselves in their suffering to be guided by cold, and as we all know, not infrequently manipulated statistics about the effectiveness of the various chemicals they are asked to ingest? What kind of rigid and inflexible worldview informs those who dismiss the hopes and concerns of that sector of the population who, for whatever reason, feel themselves inadequately cared for by this biochemical, biophysical, and technology-dominated medicine? Psychological orientation and issues of worldview play important roles in the responses of individuals to their bodily and spiritual suffering, responses that cannot be adequately captured by referring to the statistical tables of biostatisticians.

An appreciation of the historical facts might also lead to the insight that efforts to preserve and maintain for the future any traditional Chinese medicine that is anchored in ancient Chinese culture are hopeless. Just the act of sterilizing acupuncture needles removes the practice from its cultural context and implicates it with modern medicine. Whenever someone claims to be utilizing the "true, canonical" acupuncture, they are still quite unlikely to consider using dirty needles from a greasy leather or cloth binding, as was the norm only a few decades ago in China outside of the modern hospitals.

The Chinese medicine documented in the ancient medical classics owes its insights into human health and disease to the social doctrines and social and cultural environment of its creators. This environment has long faded from history, so much in ancient Chinese medicine has lost its original meaning. This is one of the reasons it is so difficult for young Chinese today to incorporate ancient concepts into their modern lives. In the end the only thing they can do, if they wish to make the effort, is to mechanically apply the old ideas. For people in Western countries wishing to use these concepts, there is an additional barrier: the language and the necessity of translating the relevant terminology.

A simple example can be used to demonstrate how even a skillful and philologically accurate translation inevitably leads to the decontextualization of the translated content. As shown at the beginning of this book, classical Chinese texts generally use the word *zhi* to denote medical "treatment," "therapy," and also "healing." The character *zhi* originally referred to the "management of irrigation" before its meaning was extrapolated to refer to the proper management of other aspects of daily life, principally political affairs and then also the body in both health and disease. Insofar as the ancient Chinese readers encountered the word *zhi* and with it, the notion of management, in both political and medical contexts simultaneously, they came to a subconscious association between the conditions under which the state was well managed and at peace, and the conditions that preserved or restored the health of the individual person.

This is not just a superficial example of parallelism. The ambivalent meaning of the word *zhi* is merely a symbol of the correspondence between political and medical concepts in the ancient academic world and lived environment. This correspondence can be found in other aspects of ancient Chinese medicine. However, it is unavoidably lost in the process of translation into Western languages. In the political context, we are required to translate *zhi* as "to rule" or "to put in order." When translating medical texts we render it as "to treat," "to medicate," or "to heal." This linguistic distinction causes us to lose sight of the social and individual nexus between political management and healing that is so important in ancient Chinese medicine. The healing/management of the human organism was indistinguishable from the healing/management of the social organism, yet through the act of translation an unavoidable division into two distinct fields is created.

Efforts to remain true to the metaphors of Chinese medical terminology in translation, to show the close correspondence of this medicine with its cultural reference points, have been repeatedly criticized by Western supporters of TCM as constituting attempts to disparage it. There is a certain paradoxical irony behind such criticism: on the one hand, TCM is supposed to be an "alternative" practice, but on the other hand, it would be better accepted if it were presented as "scientific."

Indeed it does sound rather unscientific, when one translates *feng huo yan* word for word as "wind fire eyes" instead of "acute conjunctivitis." Similarly, using the literal term "long-term depot" to translate the group of *zang* organs, and "short-term repositories" or "palaces" to translate the other organ group, the *fu*, may sound less scientific than terms that ignore the metaphorical layers of meaning of the classical Chinese, such as "full and hollow organs" or even further removed, but in classical-sounding Latin, the "*orbes functionales.*"

Within Western literature on TCM there is a general tendency to take the concrete morphological and anatomical units described unambiguously as organs in the classical medical texts and reinterpret them as "systems of function," just as there is widespread hesitation to take the Chinese terms for such objects as the liver and kidneys and translate them straightforwardly as "liver" and "kidneys." The same is true of the term "blood" in Chinese. This attitude is justified with the explanation that the functions of the organs and of the blood in ancient Chinese medical theory differ from our modern understandings.

Such a rationale is nonsensical, first of all because even the oldest texts contain exact descriptions of the organs that correspond to anatomical reality, and second because, if one were to follow this line of reasoning, it would also not be permissible to translate the Chinese words for "eyes," "nose," "ears," and so on with the corresponding modern terms in Western languages, because they represent understandings of functional integration in antiquity that are different from their functions today. To cap it all, this logic would require a refusal to consult or rewrite any European medical works from the nineteenth century because they were also informed by markedly different conceptualizations of the physiological and pathological roles of the liver, kidneys, and blood. References to such differences can in fact be deduced from the context or indicated in annotations.

Before there can be an objective discussion about Chinese medicine, other obstacles must be acknowledged. Among these are the myths that TCM is "natural, holistic, gentle, and thousands of years old." Even though these myths are deeply entrenched in Western discourse, they are not at all accurate.

The favorable attribution of TCM as "thousands of years old" is a contradiction of the historical facts. Chinese medicine could also never have been accused of being "gentle." The coarse metal pins that were thrust into the body's tissues as instruments of acupuncture had very little in common with the hair-thin, painless needle therapy of today. The letting of blood from veins, a practice that was an integral part of acupuncture for a period of several centuries, is also hardly a "gentle" procedure. The military vocabulary of medicine is another indication that "gentle" interventions were not the norm. TCM might have been legitimately referred to as a "gentle, natural" healing modality if it relied on light, the sun, warmth, the earth, and water as natural resources to exert their effects on the body, and in conjunction with the body's own natural healing forces aimed to protect and restore a person's health. There is a long history of this kind of healing modality in European countries such as Germany, but the label simply does not apply to traditional Chinese medicine and should not be appropriated by it. Chinese medical theory is influenced by China's social philosophies. Its vegetable-, animal-, and mineral-based medications are mostly drawn from the natural world, but then they are artificially changed into drug preparations that are highly culturally sophisticated, and by the same token, highly modified from their natural states. Chinese medicine does not recognize the forces of self-healing.

In the entire corpus of Chinese medical literature from the past two thousand years there is not a single discussion of the fact that many ailments resolve themselves, in spite of the fact that this was known and confirmed by Chinese observers. This phenomenon of self-healing led to recurring attempts to interpret it in the course of European medical history, but not in China. Instead, the Chinese medical authors described their medications as "soldiers" sent to wage war within the body. Physicians were thought of as the commanders leading their soldiers into war. The vocabulary that referred to such pathological events as the encroachment of one particular organ in the body on another was couched in military terms in accordance with its conceptualization as a military event.

There is no trace of this in today's Western textbooks. In the course of TCM's creative reception, it has been customized to meet the yearning of so many sensitive people in Western industrialized nations for peace and harmony; however, it cannot be said to have remained "Chinese" during this process of appropriation. In China it was a cultural product, but in its Western adaptation it is now a "systemic artifact," so to label it as "natural" is far removed from any reality.

The claim of holism drew particular attention from the civilization-jaded citizens of Western industrial nations who were consciously or subconsciously searching for a remedy for what they perceived as the increasingly splintered character of society and culture. Western medicine offers a variety of therapies that go beyond its biochemical and biophysical approaches to address the long-recognized relationship between body and soul/spirit/mind, including both psychotherapy and psychosomatics, which it deploys in the service of the prevention and treatment of disease. Chinese medicine had never put this "holism" clearly into practice. There is no term in historical Chinese medical texts for "holism"; it is a Western construct.

Inspired by this purely Western notion of holism, Western practitioners searched for a counterpart in the theory of Chinese medicine, and of course they found it. They refer to the fact that diseases in TCM are not to be treated in a localized and isolated way, but rather as disturbances of the entire organism. The assessment proceeds by noting that Western medicine is theoretically up to this challenge of holistic treatment but rarely achieves it in daily practice, a situation they compare with the holistic theory of TCM or Chinese medicine, overlooking the fact that this ideal of holistic treatment is similarly not realized in every encounter between doctors and patients in TCM, either in China or in the West.

How is it possible nowadays to call a system of medicine "holistic" when it performs no surgery and does not understand hygiene since it has no concept of viruses or bacteria? What sense does it make to denote a medicine as holistic when it only treats the individual and burdens him or her with all the blame for diseases, and is not capable of integrating lifestyle, work, or environmental risk factors as contributors to disease except in terms of such woolly concepts as yin and yang and "energetic congestion," let alone of taking the initiative to request from government the implementation of public health measures? How can a system of medicine be holistic if it does not consistently recognize the brain and the uterus as morphological units, and so has no ability to deal with either blood clots in the brain or cervical cancer?

The very definition of "holism" is hotly contested. In particular, the supposed focus of Western medicine on bodily aspects that lend themselves to biological investigation together with its disregard of "spiritual" aspects constitute a perennial inducement to represent it as the undesirable opposite of other systems of medicine that are labeled holistic because they consider the physical and the spiritual aspects as united, and do not attempt to separate soma and psyche. In this context, an important aspect is being overlooked. The secular medicine of the West is also a medicine of freedom. There are good reasons this system has a recognizable tendency to restrict itself to bodily phenomena, to the material aspects of human existence. Even though this tendency is regularly criticized, it is true to the ideal of allowing people freedom of thought. The technical term "holistic" comes from Greek. It sounds positive. But one could just as well employ the equivalent Latin term, which would be "totalitarian." This sounds much less positive, but it is a faithful indication of the danger intrinsic to this kind of medicine: its potential to exercise complete control not only over the behavior of people but also over their thoughts.

In the normal practice of conventional medicine, patients are told what they should eat and drink, how they should dress, how much to rest or to work, and how to manage their sex lives, in order to protect their health. But their thoughts remain free. In the final analysis, there is the hidden danger in a "holistic" medicine that some people will take the initiative to dictate the ideal combination of soma and psyche, with instructions for achieving the right consciousness, correct thought patterns, appropriate emotions, and so on. People who are comfortable restricting their freedoms in these ways will easily find like-minded groups, of which there are plenty enough, and work with them to find ways to overcome the limits inherent in conventional medicine. But the freedom of mind that is preserved amid the self-imposed restrictions of conventional medicine is not a good that should be surrendered lightly. In any case, TCM fails to meet the requirements of both a holism in a narrow sense limited to the body and its physical and social environment and a holism in a comprehensive sense describing a unity of body and mind.

Over the last few decades, many physicians and other health care practitioners have built their practices and written books based on such myths as have been described here, as well as others. These myths were presented to them by their teachers, included in their textbooks, and not least, promoted by the popular media. The title pages of several of the popular journals that have engaged with the theme of Chinese medicine show what symbols they use to resonate with readers and win over new ones, while simultaneously confirming their audience's prejudices. In most cases we see the image of a woman, as scantily clad as possible, suggesting a "gentle and natural" therapy. In one instance, a magazine that normally deals with primarily geological topics put its own spin on the topic of "gentle healing" with Chinese medicine by photographing a woman's naked back in such a way that it resembled, at least remotely, the kind of image of sand dunes in the Sahara that one would normally expect to see on its cover.

These myths about TCM that it is "natural, holistic, gentle, and ancient" have, in the meantime, done their duty. Even though historians consider them unjustified, they have directed the attention of large segments of the population toward Chinese medicine as an alternative to conventional medicine, and broadened the already wide spectrum of available complementary therapies.

It is now high time for an objective examination of the problematic and potential of cultural heterogeneity of health care, and the historical realities of traditional Chinese medicine. By now, there are many people participating in the clinical applications of TCM who have good to excellent knowledge of Chinese, who have studied and experienced the realities of clinical practice in China, and who run successful practices in the West. They contribute to overcoming this era of myths.

Many therapists—physicians and other health care practitioners—see quite remarkable advantages in the use of Chinese medicine. Physicians feel their professional independence to be threatened and even invalidated by the oppressive realities of the increasing commercialization of biomedical health care, expressed in terms of the requirements of insurance companies, flat-rate payments, meeting the expectations of investors, and many other pressures. They find satisfaction, on the basis of their adequately long engagement with each individual patient, in being able to broaden and expand what they see as the purely material concentration on biochemical, biophysical, and technological diagnostic and therapeutic approaches of conventional medicine with the complementary use of TCM, and this satisfaction is also transmitted to their patients.

Such patients are rarely if ever suffering from such diseases as lung embolism, fractures of the upper thigh, or breast cancer. They are mainly patients with complaints that are responsive to alternative therapeutic methods and for which they have been unable to find, or no longer believe they can find, adequate relief or cure from doctors of purely conventional medicine. An unbiased familiarity with the advantages of conventional medical approaches and with those elements of China's historical medicine that are worth retaining will perhaps facilitate a new medical culture. In this, therapies would all be measured by their contributions to the well-being of patients and not by their enforcement of biased ideologies.

EPILOGUE

It is not possible to give a single definition of "traditional Chinese medicine" either in China or in the West. Over the more than four decades since the opening of China, many different and sometimes contradictory meanings and uses of TCM have spread throughout Western industrialized nations. The multiple competing explanations of the theoretical foundations and practical clinical uses of Chinese healing are a constant reminder of the need to scrutinize our previous evaluations of its characteristics and potential.

The heterogenous contents of the rich heritage of Chinese historical works of medicine and pharmacy are only slowly being recognized. The translations of the ancient classics that began to appear in the 1970s were seldom complete and often full of errors. Because the early translators found it very difficult to render ancient Chinese concepts into modern Western languages, their versions were often characterized by the anachronistic use of modern Western terminology. As a result, it was impossible to recognize from these writings the insights that the historical authors had recorded for posterity. Only in the last few years have the most important texts of ancient Chinese medicine started to become available in

English versions that meet the normal standards of historiography and philological analysis.

Nonetheless, it is still unclear what effects these newly available sources will have on the reception of Chinese medicine in the West. The terminological approximations and cultural clichés that were coined in the 1970s have become standard usage in the intervening years. They are foundational to the identities of the many groups that are devoted to traditional Chinese medicine in the West. These identities would be threatened if the new understandings of language use and technical content were to be adopted. This makes it extremely unlikely that any homogenous system for the theory and practice of Chinese medicine will take hold in the West in the forseeable future. This would require its adherents to agree on a collective interpretation of historical theories, and just as importantly, on a standardized adaptation of Chinese terms and concepts.

To complicate matters even further, those people who went to China, the home of TCM, to study in the hope of gaining insights into authentic Chinese medicine returned with a wide variety of divergent impressions and interpretations. Disillusionment is one of the effects felt by many who return from study visits to China, partly because the situation there is also far from uniform. There are some schools that clandestinely resist—as far as is possible in China—the modern and politically motivated narrowing of historical Chinese medicine, but even though they advertise themselves to the outside world as being able to practice and teach real, authentic Chinese medicine, it is not possible for them to exclude current conditions altogether. On the other hand, anyone who observes the activities of the ubiquitous hospital enterprises, or even those who are able to get to know individual TCM doctors of excellent reputation will not infrequently be disappointed.

In the West, there is a widely held impression that "the Chinese" retain a "holistic" view of human health, and that their refined diagnostic skills are able to detect and integrate all of a person's physical and psychic states—but this impression can hardly be justified from the realities of everyday practice. Hospitals find themselves with no choice but to meet the majority of their running costs from the prescription and sale of medications. Just as is the case in many Western countries, it is often difficult to detect the boundary between medically necessary prescriptions and those primarily intended to increase the profits of their hospital administrations. The behavior of the famous doctors of TCM, whose reputations require them to deal with a constant stream of patients, is also not calculated to reinforce the idealized clichés of holistic practice that supposedly distinguish TCM from Western medicine. The fact that they conduct 100 to 150 or more consultations a day, with each patient paying a consultation fee of 50, 100, or even 200 *yuan*, is not easy to square with the images of Chinese medicine that are consistently projected in Western TCM and acupuncture courses by opponents of the industrial practices of Western medicine.

The evaluation and management of TCM is not yet a settled question on the Chinese political stage. Looking back over the past few decades, however, we can detect a significant improvement in the political valorization of China's historical medicine and pharmacy, at least in linguistic terms. This improvement correlates closely with the renewed sense of cultural pride and self-confidence that has accompanied China's growing importance as a world power.[1] For the past few years, the country has been in a fourth period of "self-strengthening," a process that it was forced to embark upon more than a century ago as a result of the scientific, technological, and medical superiority of the West. The wretched failed attempts at the end of the nineteenth century to repulse imperialist invaders with weaponry bought from them was succeeded by the second phase, consisting of a determination to study the skills and technologies from the West that were so demonstrably lacking in China. The third period is represented by the reforms introduced by Deng Xiaoping after the end of the Cultural Revolution.

Deng's opening of the Chinese market to foreign investors, with its inspired precondition that investors must form joint ventures with Chinese partners, allowed China to begin a process of technological catching up. As a result, it was only a few years before China was able to access the newest global innovations with minimal investment on its part. The results of these political developments are not only that hundreds of millions of people have been given significantly higher living standards; they also have the necessary financial means to allow the commencement of the fourth phase of "self-strengthening." China now possesses the financial resources to be able to buy up even the most expensive and prestigious high-tech companies from Western countries. In addition, China can afford to demand that any high-tech companies it has not yet acquired must reveal the technological underpinnings of their products if they want access to the Chinese market.

As a result of these policies, the newly global significance of China as an economic and increasingly also political and military power has allowed the country to gradually turn its attention back to its own culture, and to propagating this culture around the world.

Chinese medicine is also experiencing a revaluation in the course of these developments. For many years now, Chinese historians have been scouring the libraries of Japan, Europe, and other regions looking for examples of old Chinese medical texts that are no longer extant in China. When such rare texts are discovered, they are copied and republished in multivolume collected editions in China. The year 2018 will be the 500th anniversary of the birth of Li Shizhen, author of the famous encyclopedia of pharmacy and natural history. This jubilee is to be celebrated with great pomp and expenditure; already in 2016 the Chinese branch of the U.S. Discovery Channel began to prepare a multiepisode television series dedicated not only to the history of Li Shizhen but also to Chinese medicine in general.

In 2016, the Chinese cultural agency or Hanban announced a new initiative dedicated to the global dissemination and consolidation of TCM. The plan provides for the opening of a total of 200 new Confucius Institutes dedicated to TCM. The first was opened at London's South Bank University in 2015 in the presence of many honored guests. A second Institute was opened in August 2016 in Stralsund, in northern Germany. The Chinese promoters of this initiative are taking the dissemination of TCM into their own hands. It is in the Chinese interest to propagate the official Chinese version, not least in the Western industrialized nations, in order to better confront the burgeoning of idiosyncratic schools of TCM.

The political circles responsible for TCM today are no longer interested in being reminded of the opinions of Chen Duxiu, Ba Jin, Lao She, and the many other critics of a hundred years ago. The key sentences of even the "Beijing Declaration on Traditional Chinese Medicine" of 2007 would likely no longer be phrased in this way: "TCM is a form of medicine fully grounded in modern biological science," and "The future of TCM lies in molecular biology." On December 20, 2016, China's top legislature, the Standing Committee of the National People's Congress, passed a law on Traditional Chinese Medicine "to give TCM a bigger role in the medical system," to go into effect on July 1, 2017. In their identical announcements about the new law, the Chinese media emphasized that "County-level governments and above must set up TCM institutions in public-funded general hospitals and mother and child care centers. Private investment will be encouraged in these institutions. All TCM practitioners must pass tests,"[2] and "The new law puts TCM and Western medicine on equal footing in China, with better training for TCM professionals, with TCM and Western medicine learn [sic] from each other and complementing each other. The state will support TCM research and development and protect TCM intellectual property."[3]

This declaration is brimming with political rhetoric, particularly in the statement that "the new law puts TCM and Western medicine on equal footing." This formulation is vague enough to allow for all kinds of interpretation. It is nonetheless astonishing to all those who wonder how the two systems can be equally weighted when TCM is lacking in so many of the disciplines and scientific insights that are indispensable to a modern medical system.

The requirement that institutions of TCM be established at every administrative level and that private investors be found to support them suggests that TCM is to be integrated into a nationwide system of commercial medicine. Investors are entitled to demand a return on their investment. The consequences of having a health care system that promises such returns are already evident throughout the Western nations of the industrially developed world. It is hard to imagine how the ideals of historical Chinese medicine could be brought into harmony with such a system. Furthermore, the emphasis in the new law on tests to be administered to practitioners of TCM will alienate it further from its heritage. At no time in the past was "Chinese medicine" a homogenous construction of theory and practice. In fact, one of the characteristics of historical Chinese medicine was that its practitioners were at all times free to choose according to their own discretion from the multitude of ideas and practices passed down from earlier centuries. If future practitioners will now be required to pass "tests," they will have a centrally determined orthodoxy imposed on them, leading to the end of diversity. It is as yet unclear who will be responsible for specifying this orthodoxy, and what criteria are to be used to evaluate candidates' knowledge and competence.

So, even though this new law appears at first sight to enhance the status of TCM, in fact it represents an implementation of the same political line that has been followed since the founding of the People's Republic of China. The slogan that the medical systems should "learn from each other and complement each other" is a meaningful one from any standpoint. Indeed, there have been many cases where patients and their TCM doctors agree that Chinese concepts and treatments healed various ailments that Western medicine has not been able to adequately diagnose or successfully treat. The slogan is certainly not new: the requirement that the two sides should learn from and complement each other has been in frequent usage since the founding of the PRC. The same is true of the directive to investigate the historical legacy of TCM. In this case, it is clear that the "investigation" consists of nothing more than using modern scientific criteria to demonstrate the value of historical medical practices. In this way, the continued development of TCM will become completely dependent on modern physiological, pathological, and biochemical sciences.

In the course of the last few decades, many million *yuan* have flowed into the scientific investigation of acupuncture and Chinese pharmacy. This expenditure has not generally yielded the kinds of findings that would garner world attention. An exception is the discovery of an unquestionably effective antimalaria molecule in the plant *Artemisia annua* L., which with further chemical modification yields the active principle called artemisinin. A young scientist by the name of Tu Youyou, who had been educated in Western pharmaceutical research methods, was enrolled in the 1960s and 1970s in a clandestine Project 523, which was charged with the task of finding a treatment for malaria in the Chinese historical literature of *materia medica*.

This assignment was a case of looking for the needle in the proverbial haystack. The haystack was composed of the many thousands of remedies for malaria documented in innumerable writings over two thousand years, each recommending its own merits. The team, Tu Youyou among them, found ways to reduce the number of recipes for investigation to just a few hundred. Bizarre antimalaria remedies in famous historical Chinese medical works—such the recommendation to cut legendary demon tamer Zhong Kui's left leg out of pictures portraying him, reduce this scrap of paper to ashes, then ingest the ashes as medication—were understandably not included in the short list for scientific investigation. But in the course of their work, the researchers came across a text by the Daoist adept Ge Hong (284–364). In this book, titled "Recipes for Emergencies to Be Kept Close at Hand," Ge Hong had published numerous formulas, their justifications resting on the widest possible range of theories and personal experiences. In his third chapter he compiled forty-two such formulas that he declared to be helpful against malaria. The first of these had the following instructions: "Grind together pillbugs and two times seven black beans until they are evenly mixed. Ingest two pills prior [to an outbreak] and one pill at the moment [the illness] is just about to break out." The second recipe said: "A handful of *qing hao*. Soak in one *dou* of water. Wring out the juice, and ingest completely." Farther down the line are recipes based on roasted garlic, others advising one to prepare five or eight specimens of a certain type of spider, and not surprisingly in a Daoist's collection, suggestions for effective apotropaic remedies.

The researchers were interested in the recipe for *qing hao*, or *Artemisia annua*, but their first tests showed it to have only weak activity. Tu Youyou's deciding contribution was that she reread the original prescription, paying attention to its exact details. The instruction to "wring out" the drug leaped out at her: she recognized it as referring to a cold extraction. All the team's previous attempts had been with heated extracts (decoctions). When repeated with cold extraction, the tests gave the hoped-for positive results. This method evidently preserved the active principle, and further modifications led them to identify it as artemisinin. Since then, this substance has saved many lives. When Tu Youyou was awarded the Nobel Prize in 2015, there was great rejoicing in China, first of all because the prize for medicine/physiology had been awarded to someone in China. However, it soon led to a strenuous debate there as to whether the prize had been awarded to the right person.

Was the Nobel Prize an endorsement of TCM? Tu Youyou did glean information from a text that could be described as part of the heritage of historical Chinese medicine. However, Ge Hong's recipe was not influenced at all by the theoretical characteristics that make "Chinese medicine" appear so special. The likelihood that any nineteenth- or twentieth-century practitioner of Chinese medicine might have treated a patient with the cold-pressed juice of *qing hao* based on their reading of Ge Hong's fourth-century text has to be vanishingly small. So was the award of the Nobel Prize rather an endorsement of Western pharmacology? Tu Youyou's training was, in fact, in this field, and it was the methodology of Western pharmacology that guided her toward the active constituent of *qing hao* and then provided the resources to isolate and modify it into artemisinin.

Fundamentally, the award of the Nobel Prize in 2015 represents a belated reward for Mao Zedong's 1954 demand that researchers should investigate the treasure house of TCM to discover substances and techniques whose medical value could be justified with modern Western sciences. Consequently, Tu Youyou was already performing the same activities in the 1970s that are now being promoted through the new law of December 2016: that the two systems should learn from each other and complement each other. Without the instructions contained in Ge Hong's collection of remedies, modern medicine would never have discovered artemisinin, a drug that is now part of its therapeutic arsenal. But equally, without the methods of Western pharmacology, the active constituent would have remained meaningless and undiscovered, as it had been for many centuries in Ge Hong's text.

The reasoning for Tu Youyou's success is also to be found in the justification for the new law. The discovery of artemisinin is cited as evidence of the value of TCM. In fact, however, Tu Youyou's story is closer to tragedy than triumph. She, along with many other scientists in China and in other countries, has analyzed innumerable formulas looking for the possibility of similarly spectacular findings. But neither Tu Youyou nor any other researchers have been able to generate such results. One way to measure the value of TCM, as is proposed in the law of December 2016, is to look for clues in the almost infinite numbers of recipes in the ancient medical texts that will lead, after scientific analysis, to new and universally valid drugs. But this is not the main reason so many Westerners turned to this exotic healing art in the 1970s. They were looking for an alternative to the Western practice of an increasingly industrialized and commercialized medicine circumscribed by biochemistry and biophysics.

Let us take another look at what Ted Kaptchuk promised his readers back in 1983: "The Chinese physician directs his or her attention to the complete physiological and psychological individual. All relevant information, including the symptom as well as the patient's other general characteristics, is gathered and woven together until it forms what Chinese medicine calls a 'pattern of disharmony.' . . . Oriental diagnostic technique renders an almost poetic, yet workable, description of a whole person."[4] Even then, this statement failed to describe accurately the practice of historical Chinese medicine, and it is even less accurate as a characterization of the current practice of TCM in China.

Notwithstanding the actual therapeutic successes achieved with the theory and practice of today's Chinese medicine, its value for the Western public lies on two other levels. The first is the conviction that any healing system is incomplete and unsatisfactory if it relies only on statistics, algorithms, and other measurable parameters dictated by the commercial interests of its investors and pays no attention to the hopes and anxieties of real people, whether they are sick or healthy. TCM has been able to gain the trust of so many people primarily because it seemed to represent the opposite of these widespread failings of Western medicine. Even though the actual practice of TCM frequently fails to justify this confidence, its popularity can be read as a warning to take the needs and expectations of patients seriously, even while doing so is becoming more and more difficult for both Western and Chinese medicine.

A second source of the value of historical Chinese medicine, not TCM, is that it brings back into the foreground a worldview that shaped the existence of Chinese elites for two thousand years: the concept of the interrelatedness of all phenomena. The same worldview also existed for a long time in ancient Europe, although it was certainly not as consistently developed as in China, and was finally displaced in the early modern period with the rise of the analytical sciences. Now, however, in the age of information technology, it seems that the West is ready to learn to understand the "network" again. It is the network of existence within which we are all entangled. It is also the network that forms the foundation of modern technology. It is quite possible that a culture that has had the "network" constantly in mind over the last two thousand years might be able to use it to advantage again today.

NOTES

1. Origins and Characteristics of Chinese Medicine

1. The word *Gottherscher* would be more accurately translated "Thearch," god-king, but most readers will be more familiar with Qin Shi Huang Di as simply "First Emperor of Qin."
2. Harro von Senger, *Moulüe—Supraplanung: Unerkannte Denkhorizonte aus dem Reich der Mitte* ["Moulüe" or ultraplanning: unknown thought horizons from the Middle Kingdom] (Munich: Carl Hanser Verlag, 2008).

2. The Lack of Existential Autonomy

1. *Analects* book 12, number 5. Translation from Edward Slingerland, *Confucius: Analects* (Indianapolis: Hackett, 2003), 127.
2. *Shijing*, Chu ci, 楚茨.
3. *Shijing*, Chu ci, 楚茨, 209.
4. *Shijing*, part III, book 3, ode 2, *Yunhan* (Milky Way).

3. The Longing for Existential Autonomy

1. Friedrich Engels, *Anti-Dühring*, chapter 11, "Freedom and Necessity." https://www.marxists.org/archive/marx/works/1877/anti-duhring/ch09.htm.
2. *Huangdi nei jing, Su wen*, chapter 26: 血氣者，人之神，不可不謹養.

4. Quotations from the Medical Classics

1. *Huang Di nei jing su wen*, chapter 69: 邪之所湊其氣必虛.
2. *Huang Di nei jing su wen*, chapter 3: 精神內守 病安從來.
3. *Huang Di nei jing su wen*, chapter 68: 應則順否則逆 逆則變生 變則病.
4. *Huang Di nei jing su wen*, chapter 25: 天覆地載,萬物悉備,莫貴於人,人以天地之氣生,四時之法成.
5. *Huang Di nei jing su wen*, chapter 3: 謹道如法，長有天命.
6. *Huang Di nei jing su wen*, chapter 56: 上下同法.
7. *Huang Di nei jing su wen*, chapter 70: 微者復微，甚者復甚，氣之常也.

5. The Banality of Violence

1. *Huang Di nei jing su wen*, ch. 69: 氣相生者和 不相生者病.
2. *Huang Di nei jing su wen*, ch. 74: 明知勝复 為完民式 添之道畢.

8. Deficiencies in the Credibility of the New Medicine

1. Translator's comment: The German word *Fremdbestimmung* is here translated as "heteronomy," a term defined by Kant as "laws imposed from without."

9. The Alternative Model: The View from Illness

1. Michel Strickmann, *Chinese Magical Medicine*, ed. Bernard Faure (Stanford: Stanford University Press, 2012), 1ff.
2. *Qian jin yi fang*, ch. 29: 故老子曰吾所以有大患者為吾有身及吾無身吾有何患.
3. *Qian jin yi fang*, ch. 29: 由此觀之形質既著則痾瘵興焉. 靜言思之惟無形者可得遠於憂患矣. 夫天地聖人尚不能無患 況如風燭者乎.

11. Between Antiquity and the Modern Age

1. Paul U. Unschuld, *What Is Medicine? Western and Eastern Approaches to Healing* (Berkeley: University of California Press, 2009).

2. Paul U. Unschuld, *Was ist Medizin? Westliche und östliche Wege der Heilkunst* (What is medicine? Western and Eastern approaches to healing). 2nd ed. Munich: C. H. Beck, 2012.

3. Paul U. Unschuld and Jinsheng Zheng, *Chinese Traditional Healing: The Berlin Collections of Manuscript Volumes from the 16th Through the Early 20th Century*, 3 vols. (Leiden: Brill, 2012), 3: 1895–1904.

4. Ibid., vol. 3.

5. Ibid., 1947.

6. Paul U. Unschuld, *Medicine in China: Historical Artifacts and Images* (Munich-London-New York: Prestel, 2000), 54ff.

7. Zhang Zhibin and Paul U. Unschuld, *Dictionary of the Ben cao gang mu*, Vol. I: *Chinese Historical Illness Terminology* (Berkeley: University of California Press, 2015).

12. Two Medical Authors of the Ming and Qing Dynasties

1. Nathan Sivin, *Chinese Alchemy: Preliminary Studies* (Cambridge, MA: Harvard University Press, 1968), 81–122. Catherine Despeux, *Prescriptions d'acuponcture valant mille onces d'or. Traité d'acuponcture de Sun Simiao du VII siècle* (Paris: Guy Trédaniel, 1987), 15ff.

2. For the most detailed account in English, see Carla Nappi, *The Monkey and the Inkpot* (Cambridge, MA: Harvard University Press, 2009).

3. There is an extremely readable biography of Wan Quan by Barbara Volkmar: *Die Fallgeschichten des Arztes Wan Quan. Medizinisches Denken und Handeln in der Ming-Zeit* [The case histories of Doctor Wan Quan: medical thought and practice in the Ming era] (Munich and Jena: Urban & Firscher, 2007). The dates of Wan Quan's life and writings presented here are taken from information in this book.

4. Paul U. Unschuld and Jinsheng Zheng, *Chinese Traditional Healing: The Berlin Collections of Manuscript Volumes from the 16th Through the Early 20th Century*, 3 vols. (Leiden: Brill, 2012), 3: 2774–2777. Paul U. Unschuld, "Der chinesische Wanderarzt und seine Klientel im 19. Jahrhundert. Rekonstruktion eines Dialogs," in Helwig Schmidt-Glintzer (Hsg.), *Das andere China. Festschrift für Wolfgang Bauer zum*

65.*Geburtstag*, Wolfenbütteler Forschungen Vol. 62 (Wiesbaden: Harrassowitz Verlag, 1995), 129–175.

5. Nian Xiyao, *Jiyan liangfang*, preface to *Jingyan sizhong*, 1a–1b, n.d., in Paul U. Unschuld, *Medizin und Ethik. Sozialkonflikte im China der Kaiserzeit* [Medicine and ethics: social conflict in imperial China] (Wiesbaden: Franz Steiner Verlag, 1975), 65.

6. Ulrike Unschuld, "Das Tang-yeh pen-ts'ao und die Übertragung der klassischen chinesischen Medizintheorie auf die Praxis der Drogenanwendung [The *Tang-yeh pen-ts'ao* and the application of classical medical theory to the practice of pharmacy]," diss., University of Munich, 1972. Ulrike Unschuld, "Traditional Chinese Pharmacology. An Analysis of Its Development in the Thirteenth Century," *Isis* 68 (1977): 224–248.

7. When the author of this book interviewed many doctors of TCM in Taiwan during 1969 and 1970, most of whom had come to the island after the civil war on the mainland, he found the same situation to be the case. Virtually every interviewee asserted that he was the only person—with the possible exception of his own teacher—who knew how to apply Chinese medicine correctly. See Paul U. Unschuld, *Die Praxis des traditionellen chinesischen Heilsystems, unter Einschluß der Pharmazie dargestellt an der heutigen Situation auf Taiwan* [The practice of the traditional Chinese healing system, including its pharmacy, as represented by the current situation on Taiwan] (Wiesbaden: Franz Steiner Verlag, 1973). For selected quotations showing the self-representation of the interviewees, see 27–29.

8. Paul U. Unschuld, *Forgotten Traditions of Ancient Chinese Medicine: A Chinese View from the Eighteenth Century: The I-hsüeh Yüan Liu Lun of 1757 by Hsü Ta-Ch'un* (Brookline: Paradigm Publications, 1990). The quotations from Xu Dachun are taken from the preface of his work.

9. Evariste Regis Huc (1857), cited in Ralph Croizier, *Traditional Medicine in Modern China* (Cambridge, MA: Harvard University Press, 1968), 31.

10. Xu Yanzuo, *Yicui jingyan* (Guangzhou: Tieru yixian, 1896), 24a. Cited in Unschuld, *Medizin und Ethik*, 77. Croizier, *Traditional Medicine in Modern China*, 32, cites a typical critique of the avarice of English doctors of the same era: "The best cure he has done is upon

his own purse, which from a leane sickness he hath made lusty, and in flesh." Similar statements about doctors in Europe could also be cited.

13. The Confrontation with the Western Way of Life

1. Paul U. Unschuld, *The Fall and Rise of China: Healing the Trauma of History* (London: Reaktion; Chicago: University of Chicago Press, 2013).
2. Liang Qichao, "Discussing the Medical Philanthropy Society," cited in Ralph Croizier, *Traditional Medicine in Modern China* (Cambridge, MA: Harvard University Press, 1968), 60.
3. Ibid., 61. The "eight-legged essay" was the essay form required for the Chinese civil service examinations.

14. The Persuasiveness of Western Medicine

1. Wu Lien Teh, *Plague Fighter: The Autobiography of a Modern Chinese Physician* (Cambridge: W. Heffer and Sons Ltd., 1959).

15. The Opinions of Intellectuals and Politicians

1. Known in English under the title "Grandma Takes Charge."
2. Tan Zhuang 潭壯, "Dui yu zhong guo mu qian yi xue de shang tao" 對於中國目前醫學的商討, *Guo fang wei sheng* 國防衛生 10 (1941), quoted by Ralph Croizier, *Traditional Medicine in Modern China* (Cambridge, MA: Harvard University Press, 1968), 155.
3. Kim Taylor, *Chinese Medicine in Early Communist China, 1945–1963: A Medicine of Revolution* (London/New York: Routledge Curzon, 2005), 70ff., quote at 73.
4. Cited in ibid., 120–121.

16. The Selection

1. Barbara Volkmar, *Die Fallgeschichten des Arztes Wan Quan. Medizinisches Denken und Handeln in der Ming-Zeit* [The case histories of

Doctor Wan Quan: medical thought and practice in the Ming era] (Munich and Jena: Urban and Firscher, 2007), vi.

2. Jürgen Kovacs and Paul U. Unschuld, *Essential Subtleties on the Silver Sea: The Yin-hai jing-wei: A Chinese Classic on Ophthalmology* (Berkeley/Los Angeles: University of California Press, 1998), 204f.

3. Ibid., 173.

18. The Creative Reception of Chinese Medicine in the West

1. http://portal.mytum.de/pressestelle.pressemitteilungen/News Article_20110706_145242, accessed January 15, 2013.

2. Hanjo Lehman, "Akupunktur im Westen: Am Anfang war ein Scharlatan" [Acupuncture in the West: in the beginning was a charlatan], *Deutsche Ärzteblatt* 107, no. 30 (2010): A-1454/B-1288/C-1268. An extended version of this essay can be found at http://tcm.de/html/george_soulie_de_morant.html.

3. Ted J. Kaptchuk, *The Web That Has No Weaver: Understanding Chinese Medicine* (New York: Congdon and Weed, 1983), 4.

4. Ibid., 35f.

5. Manfred Porkert, *The Theoretical Foundations of Chinese Medicine: Systems of Correspondence* (Cambridge, MA: MIT Press, 1974), 161.

6. C. C. Schnorrenberger, "The Status of Diagnostics in Traditional Chinese and Modern Western Medicine," in *Physikalische Medizin und Rehabilitation. Zeitschrift für praxisnahe Medizin* [Physical medicine and rehabilitiation: a journal of applied clinical medicine] 18, no. 5 (1977): 213–219, with respect to M. Porkert, "The Scientific Place of Acupuncture," *Münchner Medizinische Wochenschrift* [Munich medical weekly] 118, no. 14 (1976): 422.

7. Manfred Porkert, *Deutsche Predigten zur chinesischen Medizin 1 und 2* [German sermons on Chinese medicine, 1 and 2] (Dinkelscherben: Phainon, 1998).

8. Beat Gerber, June 6, 2012, http://www.sciencesofa.info/2012/06/medien splitter-18-markig-mutige-worte-zur-krebsforschung-%E2%80%93-wo-bleiben-die-geschichten-dazu/, accessed January 1, 2017.

Epilogue

1. Paul U. Unschuld, *The Fall and Rise of China: Healing the Trauma of History* (London: Reaktion; Chicago: University of Chicago Press, 2013).
2. http://english.cctv.com/2016/12/27/VIDEzK2MhSUV11EXRHZ oR2gx161227.shtml, accessed February 8, 2017.
3. http://www.chinadaily.com.cn/china/2016–12/25/content _27768926.htm, accessed February 8, 2017.
4. Ted Kaptchuk, *Understanding Chinese Medicine* (New York: Congdon and Weed, 1983), 4.

INDEX

abortions, 58, 71
Acuponcture Chinoise, L' (Soulié de Morant), 124
acupuncture, 2, 27, 43, 58, 117, 123; "acupuncture mania" in Europe, 4; banned and criticized in China, 4; CIA investigation of, 115; Confucian ideology and, 62–63; creation of "New Acupuncture," 107–108; as method of bloodletting, 34, 136; scientific investigation of, 148; sterilization of needles in Western practice, 133. *See also* needle therapy
alchemy, 23, 46
"alternative" healing practices, 132
amulets, 53
Analects, Confucian, 14
anatomy, 80, 95, 113
ancestors, 12–13, 21, 23, 39, 40

anthroposophists, in Germany, 129
Artemisia annua L., 148, 149
artemisinin, 150–51
Avalokiteshvara, 51
Ayurveda, 2

Ba Jin, 101–102, 123, 146
"Beijing Declaration on Traditional Chinese Medicine," 117, 146–47
Ben cao gang mu (1593), 61, 62, 65, 71, 110
Ben cao gang mu shi yi. See Supplements to the compendium of materia medica
"Bid Farewell to Chinese Medicine" (Zhang Gongyao, 2006), 106–107
biomedicine, 116, 122, 132, 141
bladder, 31, 33, 80

blood, 17, 28, 32, 125, 135; acupuncture as bloodletting, 34; administrative hierarchy and, 30; circulation of, 95; flow of, 35

bodhisattvas, 51–52

body, human: administrative hierarchy and, 30; as governable organism, 26; self-healing of, 78–79; "warp threads" (*jing*) in, 31–32; yin-yang theory and, 31, 75

Book of Songs, The, 14–15

Boxer Rebellion (1900), 102

brain, 35, 138

breathing exercises, 27, 32, 53, 63

Britain/British Empire, 1, 88–89

British East India Company, 88

Buddhism, 25, 49–52, 55, 56; Eightfold Path, 50–51; Four Noble Truths, 50; Mahayana, 51; nirvana as true healing, 48

"Call to Youth" (Chen Duxiu, 1919), 99–100

calor innatus (innate warmth), 33–34

Chen Duxiu, 99–100, 146

Chen Yan, 126

China, 40, 108; Buddhism in, 48, 52; comparison with ancient Greece, 24; cultural heritage of, 10–11; humiliated by Japan and Western powers, 89–90, 106; modernization of, 103; "treasure ship" armada of

Zheng He, 87–88; waves of "self-strengthening," 144–45; Western students of TCM in, 143

China, People's Republic of (PRC), 4–5, 68, 102, 106, 148; "cherry-picking" political approach to TCM, 131; growing confidence as world power, 144; opening of 1970s, 104, 124, 125–26, 145; politicians and development of Chinese medicine in, 107; U.S. relations with, 115

China, Republic of, 9, 89

Chinese Imperial Medical Academy, 4

Chinese medicine, historical, 9, 18, 64, 74; ancient texts in English translation, 142–43; China's social philosophies and, 136–37; Chinese reformers' critiques of, 82, 90–91, 101–104, 123; diagnostics in, 29; emergence of, 2–3; existential autonomy and, 25; gradual suppression of, 92; individual responsibility in, 97; Internet sources of information about, 119; interrelated network of existence and, 152; literary testimony of elites and, 54; as "lost tradition," 75; medicine as *xiao dao* ("lesser way"), 77; modernization of, 103–104; origins and early history of, 27;

folk healers, 102

Formulas Organized According to the Three Types of Causes Underlying All Diseases (Chen Yan), 126

Four Elements theory, 52, 53

France, 89, 93, 99, 104, 124

fu (short-term storage organs), 18, 31, 36, 79–80, 135

gall bladder, 33

Ge Hong, 16, 22–23, 149, 150, 151

George III, King, 88

Germany, 121–22, 123, 127, 129, 136, 146

ghosts, 14–15

ginseng (*ren shen*), 45, 46

Greece, ancient, 24

Guanyin, 51–52

Han dynasty, 3, 13, 28, 38, 39, 55; as first flourishing of united empire, 76; medical substances described during, 62; new medicine of, 49

health insurance, 69, 97

heart, 33, 36, 46; as "administrative center," 30; compared to political ruler, 40; seasons and, 35

"heart envelope," 40

heaven, 14, 16; bureaucracy of, 42; earthly conditions projected into, 42; Mandate of Heaven, 22

herbal medicine, Chinese, 1

Hippocrates, 21

holism, 127, 137, 138, 139–40, 144

"hot" treatments, 57

Huang Di nei jing. See *Yellow Emperor's Inner Classic*

Huang Di nei jing tai su, 40

"Hugging a Grandson" [*Bao sun*] (Lao She, 1933), 102

India, 2, 25, 52

intestines, 33

Investigation of Drug Properties (*Yao xing kao*), 59

"invisible needle," 111

Japan, 1, 4, 40, 145; Chinese medical students in, 95, 101; German concessions in China transferred to, 99; imperialist designs on China, 89

Jesuits, 1

Jia yi jing (third century), 63

Jin dynasty, 56, 58, 61, 74, 76

Kangxi emperor, 93

Kang Youwei, 91–92

Kaptchuk, Ted, 126–27, 151

karma, 50

kidneys, 30, 33, 36, 135, 136

Kissinger, Henry, 115

Laborer's Love [*Lao gong zhi ai qing*] (film, dir. Zhang Shichuan, 1922), 101

Lao She, 102, 146

Laozi, 43, 44

law (*fa*), 22, 49
Legalism, 25, 39, 56
Liang Qichao, 91–92
Ling shu. See *Yellow Emperor's Inner Classic, Divine Pivot*
Li Shizhen, 62, 65–66, 145–46
liver, 33, 36, 135, 136; as "administrative center," 30; eyes and, 19; obstruction illnesses and, 80; seasons and, 35
Lu Xun, 100–101, 123

Macartney, Lord, 88–89
malpractice, 73, 123
"Manchurian plague" outbreak (1910–1911), 97–98
Mao Zedong, 103–104, 105, 108, 113, 150
Martianus desmestoides Chevrolat ("foreign insect"), 59
massage therapy, 34
materia medica literature, 62, 108, 148
Mawangdui manuscripts, 27–29, 43, 45; drug recipes excavated from tombs, 70; medical substances described in, 62
may apple (*lang dang*), 45, 46
medications, 28
"Medicine" [*Yao*] (Lu Xun), 100–101
meditation, 53
mental illness, 131
mercury (*shui yin*), 45, 46
Ming dynasty, 66, 71, 74, 75, 76

missionaries, American and British, 1, 94–95
Mohism, 39
Morgagni, Giovanni Battista, 80
"Morning" (Lu Xun), 101
morphology, 3, 33, 80, 95
moxibustion, 1, 63

Nan jing. See *Classic of Difficult Issues*
natural laws, 36, 37, 43, 56; existential autonomy and, 49; Mandate of Heaven and, 22; Mawangdui manuscripts and, 28
needle therapy, 34, 45, 63, 116, 123. *See also* acupuncture
Neo-Confucianism, 76
Nian Xiyao, 69
nirvana, 48–49, 51
Nixon, Richard, 115, 125

ocean tides, 36
On the Locations and Causes of Disease [*De Sedibus et Causis Morborum*] (Morgagni, 1761), 80
ophthalmology, 111–12
Opium Wars, 89
organs, 29, 137; as "administrative centers," 30–31; morphology of, 33; *qi* of, 34; seasons and, 35–36; spirits attached to, 17–18; yin-yang theory and, 31. See also *fu; zang; specific organs*
ox scapulae, divination by, 12–13

pain, 32
Parennin, Father, 93
pathology, 34, 36, 80, 113, 128, 129
Peking Union Medical College, 95
pharmaceuticals, 2, 5, 32, 132;
    counterfeit, 60; description of
    medicinal drugs, 45–47;
    elaborate technologies of, 28;
    European medicine and, 93;
    European pharmaceutical
    industry, 61; medical versus
    pharmaceutical literature, 45;
    patients killed by, 83;
    prescription collections, 70–71;
    yin-yang theory and, 43
physicians, Chinese, 28, 58, 151;
    case records of, 72–73; as
    commanders in war against
    disease, 137; disparagement of
    colleagues, 73, 156n7; employed
    by apothecary shops, 68;
    financial incentives for, 69;
    itinerant healers, 67–68, 69, 72;
    "Mr. Aconite," 56–57
physicians, European/Western, 3,
    4, 66, 68
physiology, 3, 34, 36, 113, 129
Porkert, Manfred, 127–29
Portugal/Portuguese, 1
"Posthumous Son, A" [Yi fu zi]
    (Ye Shaojun), 103
prognostication, 28
Project 523, 148–50
psychotherapy, 138
public health, 96–97, 138
Pu ji fang, 71

pulse diagnosis, 29
Pu Yi, Emperor, 9

qi, 17, 25, 79, 131; conduits of, 28,
    29, 32, 107–108, 125; congestion
    in flow of, 32; conservation of,
    21; as "energy," 119, 125, 127; evil
    or poisonous, 40, 46, 111,
    128–29; flow of, 35, 62; heaven
    and earth as sources of, 22;
    importance in therapeutics, 34;
    Internet sources of information
    about, 119, 121; as material
    substance, 23; stored in organs,
    18; as superstition, 100; "visitor
    qi" (ke qi), 128
Qi Bo, 20–21, 39
Qin dynasty, 3
Qing dynasty, 63, 66, 74, 82
Qin Shi Huang Di ("First
    Emperor of Qin"), 9–10, 12,
    153n1 (ch. 1)

Recipes for Emergencies to
    Be Kept Close at Hand
    (Ge Hong), 149
Reston, James, 115, 125
Rockefeller Foundation, 95

science, 24, 90, 94, 102, 120, 125;
    Chinese reformers and, 82,
    99–100, 106; indigenous
    healing arts of China and, 91;
    "Manchurian plague" outbreak
    and, 97; TCM's move away
    from, 130

seasons, 22, 25, 32, 35–36
self-healing, 79, 137
sexual practices, 27–28
shamans, 41, 42
Shang dynasty, 13
Shang han lun (Zhang Ji), 75
Shen Nong, Emperor, 118
Shen nong ben cao jing, 45–46,
    75
Sino-Japanese War (1895), 90
smallpox, 69–70
social Darwinism, 91
Society for Medical Welfare, 91
Song dynasty, 43, 56, 58, 61, 68, 82;
    herbals of, 62; officials and
    literati of, 75; theoretical
    innovations during, 74, 76
Soulié de Morant, Georges,
    124–25, 127
Soviet Union, 104
spells, 53
spirits, 13–15, 40; emotions and,
    18; "essence" and, 21; evil
    spirits as enemies, 42; as
    perpetrators of diseases, 27;
    power relations with humans,
    17, 18; rejection of superior
    power of, 16
spleen, 30, 33, 35–36, 57, 111
Sun Simiao, 43–44, 48, 65, 70, 77,
    111
*Supplements to the compendium of
    materia medica (Ben cao gang
    mu shi yi)*, 59
systematic correspondence, 45, 56,
    108, 110

Taiwan, 113, 156n7
Tang dynasty, 39, 55, 58, 65, 82
Tan Zhuang, 103
Tao Hongjing, 16, 22, 62
TCM (Traditional Chinese
    Medicine), 1–2, 4, 55, 66, 141,
    156n7; as "alternative"
    practice, 116, 135, 151; as
    "artificial systematic product,"
    107, 116; as belief system, 130;
    Chinese government
    initiatives to promote, 146–47;
    contradictions between
    Western medicine and, 80;
    difficulty of defining, 142;
    disillusioned Western
    students of, 143; handwritten
    manuscripts, 58–60;
    integrated into Western
    biomedical framework, 5;
    Internet sources of
    information about, 117–23;
    introduction of term, 104;
    modernization of, 117; as
    mythology, 112–13, 124–25, 136,
    140; Nobel Prize and, 150;
    partisan sects within, 129;
    science and, 125, 146;
    theoretical underpinnings of,
    38; training for students of,
    113; worldwide spread of,
    104–5, 142
"three burners" (*san jiao*), 34
Three Dosas theory, 52
tortoise plastrons, divination by,
    12–13

Traditional Chinese Medicine. *See* TCM (Traditional Chinese Medicine)

translation, Chinese medical terminology in, 134–35

Treatise on the Origin and Development of Medicine [*Yi xue yuan liu lun*] (Xu Dachun, 1757), 75, 81–82

tui na (push-and-pull) massage therapy, 34, 63

Tu Youyou, 148–51

"Twenty-One Demands," 89

underworld, 13, 40, 41, 42

United States, 4, 89, 95, 115

violence, normality of, 25, 43

Virchow, Rudolph, 3, 94

Volkmar, Barbara, 107

Wang Bing, 39

Wang Daxie, 98

Wan Quan, 66–75, 77, 83

Warring States period, 9, 13, 19, 25

Way, the (*dao*), 22, 42

weather, 36

Web That Has No Weaver, The (Kaptchuk), 126

Western (European) medicine, 2, 5, 55, 64; anesthetic methods as first revolution in, 93; biographies of individual physicians, 66; *calor innatus* (innate warmth) notion, 33–34; Chinese encounter with, 18, 82, 91, 92, 101; combined with Chinese medicine, 104, 105, 106; dissemination in China, 4; Doctrine of the Mean, 95; "holism" and, 137–38, 144; identified with imperialism, 103; industrial practices of, 144; missionaries and, 94–95; shortcomings of, 116, 123, 152; TCM compared with, 123–24, 146–47

World War, First, 99

writing system, Chinese, 10

Wu Lien-teh, 97–98

xie (evil, improper, heterodox), 19, 50

Xu Dachun, 66, 75–83

Xu Qiu, 75

Xu Yanghao, 75

Xu Yanzuo, 83

yangchong ("foreign insect") fad, 59

Yang Shangkun, 105

Yang Shangshan, 40

Yellow Emperor (Huang Di), 20, 39, 118

Yellow Emperor's Inner Classic (*Huang Di nei jing*), 21, 23, 36, 40, 43, 79; ailments listed in, 32–33; "Plain Questions" edition, 20, 38; as revered "ancient" text, 77; unknown authors of, 39